KindTouch® *Massage*

D1532541

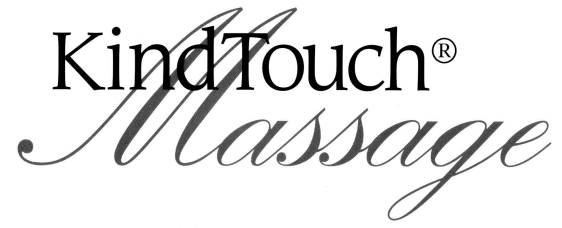

KindTouch® Massage

Self-Massage
For Health and Well-Being

Lynne Walters, RN, LMP

Photography by Kathleen M. Webster

Sterling Publishing Co., Inc.
New York

CONNETQUOT PUBLIC LIBRARY
760 OCEAN AVENUE
BOHEMIA, NEW YORK 11716
Tel: (631) 567-5079

For Joel
and to the memory of James, Marian,
and Michael Batchelor, and Billie Talley

Edited by Diane Asay
Cover and text design by Guy Boster

Library of Congress Cataloging-in-Publication Data

1   3   5   7   9   10   8   6   4   2

Published by Sterling Publishing Company, Inc.
387 Park Avenue South, New York, N.Y. 10016
© 2002 by Lynne Walters
Distributed in Canada by Sterling Publishing
c/o Canadian Manda Group, One Atlantic Avenue, Suite 105
Toronto, Ontario, Canada M6K 3E7
Distributed in Great Britain and Europe by Cassell PLC
Wellington House, 125 Strand, London WC2R 0BB, England
Distributed in Australia by Capricorn Link (Australia) Pty Ltd.
P.O. Box 704, Windsor, NSW 2756, Australia
Printed in China
All rights reserved

Sterling ISBN 0-8069-1543-9

PRECAUTIONS

Self-massage as presented in this book is safe for most conditions. Its emphasis on gentle exploration, on listening well to your body's responses, and on decreasing pressure when you find any tenderness will help you stay safe as you massage yourself. However, there are some general precautions that are good to keep in mind.

Any pain, strain, illness, infection, or injury needs to be evaluated by your doctor, who will help you determine the most effective treatments. Ask about massage therapy as a therapeutic tool. See Chapter Twelve, the section on Staying Whole, for self-massage guidelines for new injuries. Get professional massage therapy for treatment of injuries, pain that radiates from a central area, or in the presence of illnesses such as cancer, heart problems, circulatory problems, or swelling. Vigorous massage can make you feel worse if you have a cold or flu, so keep it gentle.

There are areas of the body where deep pressure must be avoided. Many are "soft spots" next to bones or joints, where you can press down into a soft depression or hollow. Often there are nerves or blood vessels running under these soft spots that can be damaged by pressure aimed down into the hollow.

Avoid applying pressure to these areas, especially when the joint is bent:

- Throat (leave this to a professional massage therapist)
- Above and below your collar bones
- The spot just below the center of the base of your skull (between the two large muscle attachments just to the sides of this hollow)
- The inside and lateral side of your upper arms where no muscles lie over the bone (and nerves and blood vessels)
- The "crazy bone" dip between the bones on the inside of the elbow
- Inside of the bent elbow, hip (groin or top of inner thigh), knee, or arm pit
- Both sides of the heel, just below the ankle bones
- The center of your buttock
- Abdomen, or over kidneys (just above and below your lowest ribs)

KindTouch Massage: Self-Massage for Health and Well-Being

Acknowledgments

Much to my surprise, it does take a village to write a book, especially one such as this. There are many people to thank, who gave generously to help this project emerge into a book.

I am indebted for the support of my self-massage group: Shirley Ferris, Jan Dorn, Richard Vaughan, Moira Gray, and Kathleen Webster. Your wisdom and healing are reflected in these pages, as well as your practical advice.

Thanks to Kathleen Webster, an extraordinary photographer, gifted in illuminating the spirit in all of us through her photography. You have been a good companion in a huge undertaking.

To Tess Taft, a great friend and inspiration, thanks from my heart for our weekly phone sessions that helped to keep this first time author sane and to bring out the gifts in this book.

My thanks to Melissa Frykman-Thieme and Doug Thieme for your open-hearted healing music.

I extend my thanks to my women's sacred circle for your belief in me, for reminding me of my wholeness when I lose sight of it, and celebrating with me when I am full of strength. Judith Parker, Barbara Snodgrass, Melissa Frykman-Thieme, Gina Marie Moy, Margaret McKinstry, Debi Cekosh, and Lorelle Parker, you are all full of life and healing power.

My gratitude goes to Shannon Seath Meyer, my colleague and friend, whose massages kept me, and the massage therapy business, going strong when I was knee deep in writing.

To my editor, Diane Asay, who helped me find and express the wisdom hidden in me, I give my gratitude. You held the overall spirit of the book and kept the details together.

All the models in this book are real people—not a professional model in the bunch. You are all gorgeous! Thanks for your generosity in sharing a visual image of the beauty, kindness, and wisdom that reside in each of us. Thank you to Barbara and DeLos Snodgrass, Tom Wilkins, Melissa Frykman-Thieme, Nan McGehee, Nancy Wing, Pam Miskimmon, Paula Hendricks, Anne Herfindahl, Richard Vaughan, Shirley Ferris, Moira Gray, Jan Dorn, and Joel Walters.

I am grateful to all my clients over the years. You kept me growing along with you.

Thanks to my friends who read the manuscript and gave realistically helpful suggestons. You saved me from many blunders. Juli Morser, Paula Hendricks, Pam Miskimmon, Shirley Ferris, Jan Dorn, Anne Herfindahl, Moira Gray, Susan Tower, and Billie Talley.

I'm grateful for my professional education and grounding. I appreciate my graduate studies at the University of Washington School of Nursing, where I focused on gerontological nursing—the study of growth and change over the adult life span. I give special thanks to Pauline Bruno, the professor who encouraged me to explore holistic health care. For massage therapy, I thank the Heide Brenneke School of Massage in Seattle, Paul St. John for his development and training in Neuromuscular Therapy, and Michael Mann's instruction in Myofascial Release. My bodywork grew from these foundations. Marty Rossman, MD, and David Bresler, PhD, founders of the Academy for Guided Imagery, gave invaluable instruction in interactive guided imagery, for my own growth as well as the ability to help others discover their own wisdom and truth through imagery. Robin Goff, a holistic nurse and minister, introduced the idea of a spiral image of healing and wholeness in a workshop at the 1999 American Holistic Nurses' Association (AHNA) Conference. The AHNA inspires me as the standard bearer for a holistic approach to nursing care.

Thank you to Shirley and Bill Ferris for giving me writing weeks at your cabin, and to Joan and Jon Hanna for your generosity in allowing us to use your beautiful studio for the photographs.

To my husband, Joel, my heartfelt gratitude for a life partner who supports me wherever my path takes me, even into writing a book.

And to you readers, who will make your own path as you move through this book, I send blessings on your journey.

Foreword

All healing that does not come spontaneously from nature or grace begins with awareness. A healing process that for whatever reason has not been able to proceed naturally can often be stimulated by the simple act of bringing loving attention to the area and allowing it to dwell there for a while. When that attention is delivered through the touch –especially the touch of a beloved – the body relaxes, and relaxation often allows healing to take place.

Relaxation allows the blood to flow more freely, and delivers important nutrients and cells of repair to the muscles. It also helps to wash away painful products of inflammation and constriction. When muscles relax, it turns down the alarm signals that the nerves send all through the body, and allows the mind to relax and become relatively quiet. When the body and mind are both quiet and at ease, Mother Nature is able to do her healing work without distraction.

Our bodies, like most living things, respond positively to attention given with tenderness, kindness and love. The body is highly intelligent, the current version of a living creation that dates back at least several billion years on earth. It is designed to survive, and to heal from injuries and wounds, whether those wounds are physically or emotionally induced. When we can approach the body with respect and trust, it will share with us the remarkable knowledge it has about healing. When it is given opportunities to feel and express what it is feeling in movement, sounds, breath, and images, it can more fully participate in healing itself.

In medicine, if we pay attention to the mind/body connection at all we usually do it through the use of the mindful skills of relaxation, imagery. meditation and related techniques. Here, you will learn to use the true native language of the body, the language of touch and movement, combined with the powerful expressive medium of imagery, to welcome the body to not only release pain and stress, but to express its joy and ability to heal.

Touching wounds and painful areas, even with attention, can hurt, so they must be touched with gentleness and tenderness. This gentleness and tenderness tells us we are safe at that moment, and, perhaps even more importantly, that we are cared for.

In the truly beautiful work that follows, Lynne Walters will guide you through gentle yet deep processes that will help you attend to yourself in a loving and deeply nourishing way – through the combined media of your own touch coupled with your own sensibility and care. Learning to be both giver and receiver of such healing attention can be a powerful stimulus to better health and an improved sense of well-being.

Beautifully conceptualized and designed, this book and the guided explorations on the CD that accompany it, are a significant contribution for all of us who believe that better caring for the self is ultimately the most effective form of true health care.

Martin L. Rossman, M.D., Dipl. Ac. (NCCAOM)
Co-Director, Academy for Guided Imagery
Mill Valley, CA 11/5/01

KindTouch
Massage

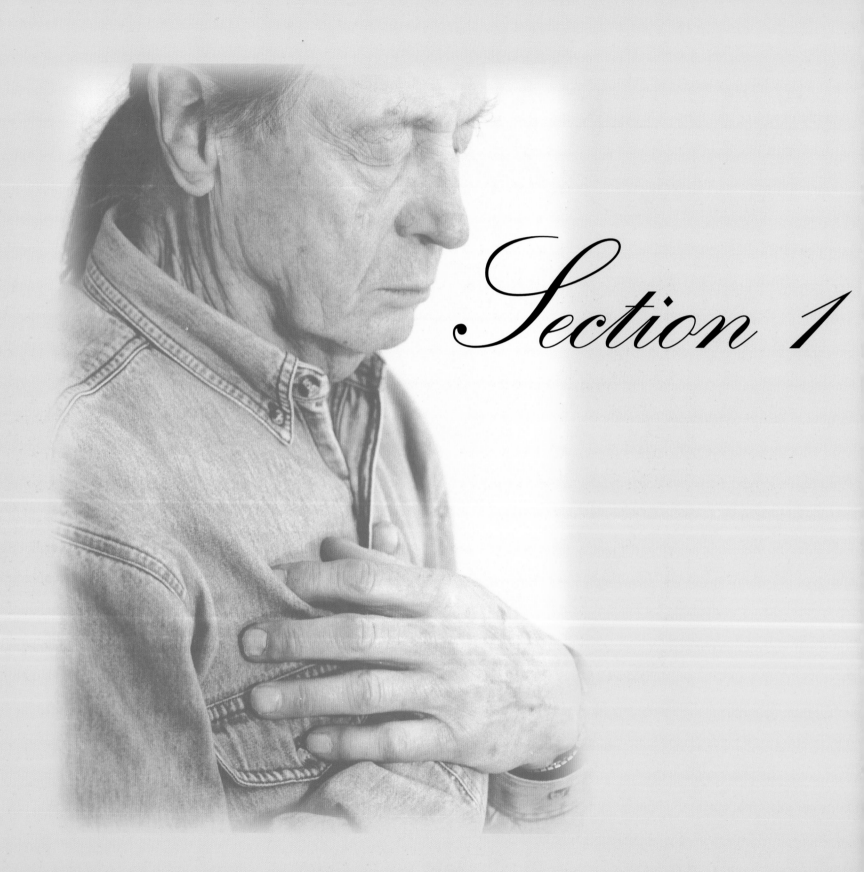

Section 1

Opening the Door to Wholeness

elf-massage can open the door to wholeness. It offers many gifts to us and softens not only our bodies but also our hearts, minds, and souls. Kind touch gives us a healing path, helping us to move toward greater wholeness. Self-massage teaches us the gentle language of kind touch, for ourselves and also for those we care about. Massaging ourselves develops our ability to listen to the messages held in our bodies, both physical and emotional. Attending to these messages furthers our healing journey. We become more able to relate to ourselves with love and compassion, and to offer forgiveness to ourselves. We learn how to reclaim parts of our bodies with which we have lost touch or that we have rejected. We find that health and illness are not opposites but merely different steps on a healing spiral, where each experience moves us further along the path. Finally, our bodies become the ground where we can embody Spirit and have a grounded, Spirit-filled experience.

...what people do to make peace with their bodies may be startlingly similar to what they do to heal their hearts.

Marc Barasch

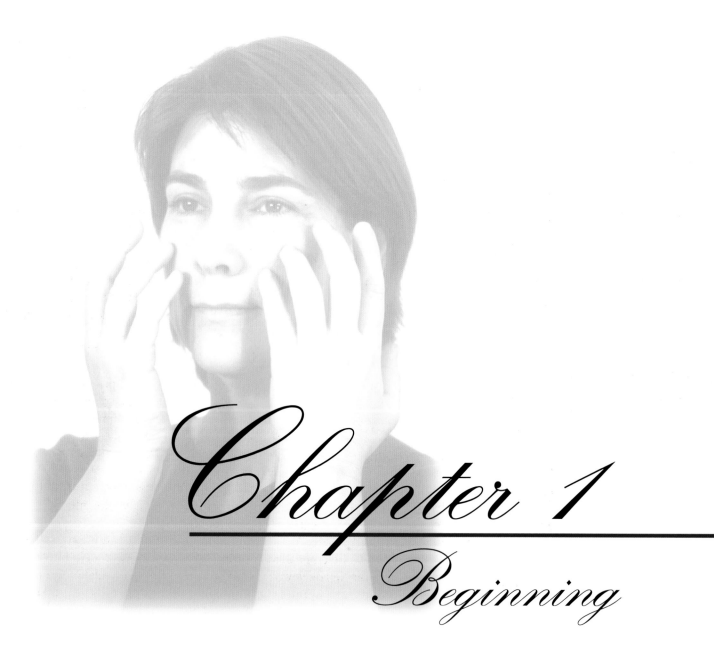

Chapter 1

Beginning

For disease confronts us with a paradox: To reclaim what we have lost, we have to use what we may not know we already possess. We have visibly fallen apart, yet to become whole again, we must bring our whole self–heart, mind, body, and spirit–to the task or recovery. Healing, as shamans have long maintained, is the business of soul retrieval.

Marc Barasch

T here's nothing better than getting a great massage from a massage therapist you know and trust. Well, there are one or two things that are better, but I can never remember what they are when I'm getting a wonderful massage! Self-massage does not replace massage therapy. It adds another dimension to your life, teaching you how to listen to your own body-wisdom, and how to treat yourself with loving-kindness. It offers the means to soften to your whole self and expand your experience of wholeness. It supports healing and helps you to have more fun taking care of yourself. Self-massage brings us into deep connection with ourselves. Working kindly with our bodies helps to heal our spirits as well as our bodies. Used in this way, it becomes soul work.

My Story

This book is a work of my heart. It has been a healing journey with great gifts that I want to share with you. It grew out of a synchronistic meeting with my editor and a lifelong career of helping others to heal. Thirty-two years of nursing, fourteen years of massage therapy, and my own experiences with some chronic conditions have given me first-hand understanding about returning to wholeness after that wholeness is threatened. I want to begin by telling you some of my story and how self-massage became a means to the experience of wholeness for me.

When I was thirteen I had major surgery to correct scoliosis, a sideways curvature of my spine. The surgeons fused eight vertebrae in my upper back, a very long fusion, leaving no movement in that area. After that surgery the curvature extended downward a few more vertebrae, but I declined the surgeon's offer of a second surgery. I still have quite a curve and rotation of my spine along with the challenges that come from having so many vertebrae fused. Since there is no movement at all in part of my upper back, all bending has to

come from my low back and neck. This puts extra stress on these areas, making them prone to pain and muscle spasms. Consequently, I have had on-and-off low back pain and muscle spasms from the time I was twenty-three.

It took a long time to work through my feelings about the violence of the surgery, which I intuitively felt had tacked down my heart chakra (one of the seven major energy centers in our bodies). I had spent a year in a body cast that went from the top of my head down to the tops of my legs so I could just barely sit. I had been burned in the groin by the "perfectly safe" saw they used to cut and shape the cast. The surgery was done at a specific point in puberty to take advantage of my spine's growth, which made for a tough beginning of adolescence. When I started having back pain as an adult, I had to relive that experience several times to work through my feelings of trauma and to release my heart chakra.

As I got older, all the doctors' predictions that things would get worse with age seemed to be coming true. I had constant back and neck pain that restricted my activities, and at the same time I had what was initially diagnosed as overuse syndrome tendinitis in both wrists and both elbows. In addition, I was tired all the time.

After two or three years I was finally diagnosed with fibromyalgia, a condition involving a lot of pain around many joints and chronic fatigue. The pain was difficult to handle, but the hardest part for me was the exhaustion. It was like no other fatigue I had ever felt; nothing like the somewhat pleasant weariness I'd felt after back packing. I had always been able to work a little harder or do a little more to get everything done, and now I could not even do the most basic work. I could do only two massages a day (my usual was four or five) and fix dinner. If I did anything else, like going out to lunch with friends,

Chapter 1 – Beginning

I had to drop one of the massages. I could no longer earn my value in the world through what I did. It was another hard lesson in learning that my value comes from who I am, not what I produce.

After the diagnosis of fibromyalgia, I was relieved finally to know what was going on and to find treatments that helped. These treatments included acupuncture, medications, very gentle massage, and learning the lessons fibromyalgia brought to me. It taught me that much of my self worth came from doing a good job "fixing" other people's problems. It was very hard for me to stop working and make taking care of myself a priority; I wanted to keep up appearances. I finally had to give up the intense way I was doing massage therapy. I had built a very successful practice based on a strenuous style of massage. It was hard to let go of this, but I found a gentle way of working with the body that affected the deep tissues just as well as the strenuous style that was so hard on my body. It has led me to a kinder way of treating both my clients and myself. Now I invite muscles to soften, instead of trying to make them change.

Following the path of listening to my body and consciously attending to its messages has deepened and broadened not only my mortal, physical self, but my spiritual self as well—my connection to Spirit. In this book I refer to God, Allah, the One, the All as "Spirit." I hope that term elicits for you the essence of your own connection with the divine as it does for me.

Looking back, I am aware that I knew early on what the pain in my hands and arms was telling me: I was working too hard to help people who were looking for an outside "fix" for their problems. This contradicted what I believed about healing and the need for softness and acceptance of ourselves in the moment. We are healed not by others, but by ourselves, often with the help of others (friends, doctors, or therapists).

A massage therapist can easily fall into a fix-it role; the client brings "the problem" and "gives it to me to fix." It is a seductive role; when things go well clients think I am great and we are all happy. But when they do not go so well there is a tension that includes an underlying unspoken question: "Whose fault is it?" Please understand! There can be no fault in healing work; there is only the path of healing.

I needed to find a way of working that included all of me as well as all of my client—our bodies, minds, hearts, and souls—working together in partnership. Things work so much better when the client and the massage therapist work together as partners, with the client in control of his or her own body and identity. It is a partnership even when it looks like one person is giving and the other is simply receiving. The ability to receive is a powerful aspect of this partnership. The massage therapist has expertise about the muscles and the therapies that can help injured tissue; but the client is the healing organism, the whole person who integrates the massage. Connecting with your whole self through self-massage will develop your ability to deeply receive the benefits from a professional massage.

In self-massage we learn how to receive what we give to ourselves. We discover the ways our own bodies respond best, and we learn how to participate more consciously in the healing process. Some of the exercises in this book reflect experiences that helped me to heal. I consider myself healed from the fibromyalgia I had for so long, but it's something I face again whenever I get over stressed and don't get enough rest. Healing is an ongoing, lifelong process. It teaches me to listen and treat myself kindly. Of course, each of us has some lessons we need to learn over and over; chronic illness can be a great teacher and reminder of those lessons. Now that I have normal energy levels again and much less pain, I realize I am still vulnerable to fibromyalgia. My body reminds me that I need to take good care of myself continually. I have learned to listen for the soft voice of mild "symptoms" and to change my ways before I fall back into that awful level of pain and fatigue again. That is one of the lessons I learned from my friend, fibromyalgia.

Using This Book with Your Massage Therapist

I highly recommend that you arrange to receive a couple of massages early in your process of reading this book. They will help you become more attuned to how your body experiences relaxation and comfort, and how massage affects tight or tense muscles. Getting a massage will also give you an experience of simply receiving, without focusing on giving or doing anything other than allowing your body to enjoy kind touch. Just let your focus rest on the massage therapist's hands and how your muscles are responding. You can also place your attention on the moment your muscles (and your whole self) shift from tension to relaxation. Once you experience these sensations, you can begin to remember them and invite these relaxed feelings back whenever you start to feel tense. Later, when you are learning how to do the massage strokes, you might want to get another massage so you can recognize how these strokes feel when given by someone who has practiced them a lot.

You can use this book as a powerful tool in conjunction with ongoing massage from a professional therapist. Your own internal work and awareness will magnify the benefits from receiving massage therapy for healing an injury, chronic pain, or restriction. You will be able to continue being present and kind to yourself and your injury in the time between massage appointments, which will improve your healing process. Learning to open to and

fully receive a massage from a therapist will expand your learning in all the areas addressed in this book.

Structure of the Book

First: a word about style. I write the same way I talk, so I'll be saying "we" and "you" throughout the book. When I say "we," I don't mean to say that my words apply to everyone; each of us is different. When I use "you," I'm often making suggestions for you to try out to see if they fit. Take what has meaning for you and move past anything that doesn't.

Section I: *Opening the Door to Wholeness* introduces you to self-massage. The second chapter discusses the benefits of self-massage more fully and includes some exercises to get you started, including the *Self-Blessing* exercise on the *KindTouch CD* and a cornerstone of this book. In chapter 3, I introduce my image of healing, the healing spiral.

Section II: *Learning the Language of Touch* will introduce you to many of the strokes used in basic massage therapy, adapted to self-massage. Once you feel comfortable with them, you will be able to massage your painful or stiff areas, and take care of yourself, and others, in a new way. Learning the strokes is only one part of massage. Equally important, you must learn how to apply them—whether to use a soft, general touch or a more focused, specific contact. This understanding will enable you to respond appropriately to the same area under different circumstances. You won't always approach one area of your body in exactly the same way; rather you will learn to listen to your muscles to discover what they need in that moment, noticing if they are soft or tight, relaxed or stiff, comfortable or tender. In short you will learn to listen and respond to your body through your hands. Chapter 9 and the second exercise on the *KindTouch CD* lead you through a guided self-massage where you will practice what you are learning in this section.

Georgia's Story

I wondered if the self-massage would feel as thorough and relaxing as receiving a massage. What I experienced was very different, something very self-contained. My hands felt larger than life. My fingers also felt very long, but very supportive, almost structural, woven together like a strong open-weave basket. My overriding sensation was one of being held in a container. I was holding and at the same time I was being held—all of my senses were in both places at the same time. Having both feelings simultaneously felt perfectly natural. It felt secure and firm and sure—a feeling of immeasurable comfort and oneness.

> *The body becomes the wisdom to understand what we need to do in terms of our healing journey.*
>
> Clyde Ford

Photographs and descriptions of strokes and exercises combine to help you learn how to create and give yourself a personalized massage.

Section III: *Moving Into Healing* explores the benefits of self-massage in depth. Each chapter includes self-exploration and self-massage exercises for you to do, and journal suggestions for you to record your experiences and keep track of key discoveries. It will be important to keep a record of the strokes and the type of touch that works best for you. This way you can pay attention to anything that changes or deepens as you work through the book. Guided imagery exercises are included to further deepen your relationship to your body. You may want to listen to my voice leading these exercises presented on the *KindTouch CD* enclosed inside the front cover, or you can record them in your own voice if you prefer. The text of the four guided imagery exercises can be found in the appendices.

You can approach the exercises as deeply as you want. You can choose to spend as little as ten minutes, or an hour or more. If your current priority is to get an overview of the path to wholeness offered in this book, you can choose to spend a shorter time with each exercise, noting the ones that speak most strongly to your own path. Then as you plan how to integrate what you learn from the book into your daily life in Chapter 13, *Grounding Spirit,* you can delve more deeply into the exercises you have chosen. Your self-massage journal will help you keep track of decisions and discoveries you make along the way. On the other hand, if your goal is to open deeply to each experience offered through the book, you can take as much time as you want. Each exercise can hold as much depth of exploration as you desire. You can devote a week to each one if you want. The exercises simply offer a route to explore your own process and experience.

In this book you will learn to follow your intuition, the power within you to know what is needed. You will use your mind and its power to visualize, by following guided imagery exercises to soften into the experience of wholeness. You will learn the strokes of massage therapy and experience the power of your deepest nature to stimulate the healing resources of your body. You can create a self-massage approach just right for you.

As you learn to listen to and massage your body, you may encounter stored tensions from past experiences as well as the tensions from the day. The more you can open to these, soften into them, and offer yourself the language of KindTouch described in this book, the more you will uncover the powerful resources for healing and joy that lie within you. If troublesome memories of past trauma surface, get support from family, friends, or a counselor to strengthen your healing journey.

I hope that your experiences through this book will help you continue to build, with power and grace, your own healing path. Connecting with your body in a way that uses the best of your mind, your heart, and your soul will bring you many gifts. I encourage you to treat your journey through this book with love and liveliness and with a sense of discovery and play.

Chapter 2
The Gifts of Self-Massage

In the midst of our hectic pace many of us lose touch with our bodies' messages. We simply want our bodies to be quiet and do whatever it takes to accomplish all that we must do. Sooner or later this approach stops working. Our bodies stumble and remind us that we need to pay attention to the practical side of living in a body. In my massage practice, I see a lot of clients so out of touch with their bodies that their pain finally has become so bad they can't ignore it anymore. They feel separate from the problem, or that the problem is separate from them, and they just want it to go away. They want me to take it away, so that they can get on with their lives. But healing involves much more than that.

We have to take responsibility for our own health. Self-massage expands our ability to do this. Through self-massage we begin to learn about our own bodies, to listen to our bodies' wisdom and to respond appropriately. We learn to relax and to soften into our wholeness. We expand our experience of wholeness when we contact and embrace hidden pain or emotions, forgive ourselves, and learn to give and receive self-love. Further healing occurs in self-massage when we focus kind touch directly on injuries or chronic conditions. Through self-massage we also begin to discover what it means to embody Spirit.

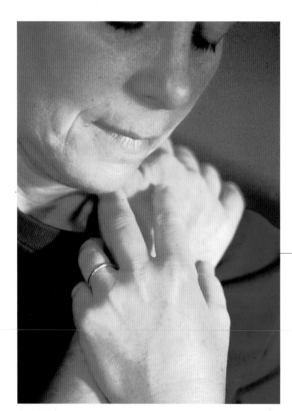

Learning the Language of Kind Touch

Learning to give yourself a sensitive massage begins by becoming comfortable doing each stroke. Many people feel they don't know how to give a massage to anyone else, much less to themselves, simply because they don't know the massage strokes. We tend to defer to experts, and may feel that massaging ourselves offers less value than receiving a massage from someone else. It's true that when we get a massage we can let go and take it all in, because we're not doing any of the physical work. But it is worth the effort to learn how to massage yourself. The strokes and the way they are used become the vocabulary of touch, and you can develop a language of touch that is unique to you.

After you learn the strokes in Section 2, you can begin to listen to what your body needs, and apply the strokes in response to the messages your body sends. You are the one who knows from the inside how you feel and what you need. It takes practice and attention to learn to give and receive at the same time, but once you can, you'll be able to bring focused, healing touch whenever you are injured or ill, and give deep support to your healing.

You can try an experiment right now. Notice an area of your body that feels stiff or uncomfortable. Then place one or both hands over it, and simply rest them there for a moment while you place your kind attention there. Notice how that area feels with this kind of focus. Then use your whole hand to make long smooth strokes over the general area, first softly, and then with more pressure, noticing what happens. Now knead the area between your fingers and the palm of your hand. Next, place your fingertips in the center of the area and press into the muscles with gentle or firm circles or a back-and-forth motion. Finish by repeating the long smooth strokes.

You've just done a version of four strokes in massage: holding, gliding, kneading, and friction. There's more to each stroke, but this can give you an idea of how it feels to massage yourself. How does the area that you just massaged feel now compared to before you started? If it feels better, you've felt a beginning benefit of KindTouch. If it doesn't feel better, you will learn in this book how to use the messages from your body to use strokes that do help.

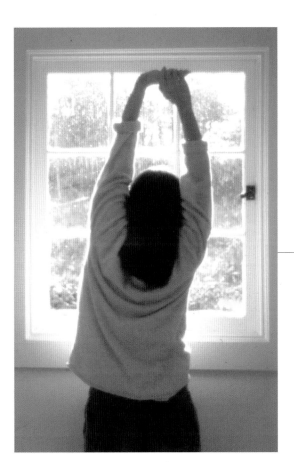

Listening to Your Whole Self

Listening

A lot of people don't know how to connect with themselves, or feel they don't have the time to do it. As babies and toddlers we experienced ourselves whole. We expressed our emotions and our needs directly through our bodies. When we were unhappy, hungry, or physically hurt we cried or screamed and stiffened our bodies. When we were happy, delighted, or felt good physically we laughed and gurgled and waved our arms and legs. Then as we grew up we gradually learned to restrict our wholehearted and whole body expressions and to limit our demands for instant satisfaction. We learned to defer gratification, to use words to express what we want, need, and feel and to be tactful and aware of others' needs as well as our own. In becoming socialized, most of us lost contact with our bodies' messages, buried our emotions, or neglected ourselves as whole beings. We lost the ability to listen to our bodies and recognize the inherent wisdom that lies within us.

Softening

It's time to get to know yourself from the inside again, and soften into acceptance of yourself as you are. You can bring your maturity and insight to the process of remembering yourself, becoming more true to yourself. You can start by merely noticing how your body moves in space and what that feels like. Listening to your body is not about what you think your body feels or what you think it should feel.

Take a minute right now to stretch with awareness. Stretch like a cat or a dog. Pay attention to how each part of your body feels during this stretching movement. Notice where you feel terrific and where you feel bound up or stiff. Does the stretch completely ease the areas that feel stiff? Do some spots return to the same level of discomfort or even feel more uncomfortable? If you notice an area that feels no relief, gently bring your attention there in a curious, "listening" state. Ask how (and if) it would like to move. Slowly begin that movement, listening all the time to your body's wishes and adjusting your movement in response. Just move in response to what gives a gentle improvement in comfort. Perhaps this area does not want to move or stretch; maybe it wants to be held and cradled, or to be gently stroked or massaged. This process of listening to your body and adjusting your touch in response begins to make you an ally with that stiff or painful part of yourself. Rather than rejecting it, or forcing it into complying with your need for it to move, you have begun to reincorporate it into your experience of who you are. The physical sensations in your body are messengers of the truth that resides within you.

Recently I was reminded that this kind of acceptance and love is a process, not an accomplishment. In the last few years I have had pain and stiffness in my neck. I worked hard to help it by stretching, exercising, and focusing on good posture. But my neck continued to hurt and be very stiff. It wasn't until I talked to my neck through imagery (as in Exercise 12e: *Talking With Your Pain*, the last guided exercise on the *KindTouch* CD) that I learned something that revolutionized my relationship with this part of myself. I received a simple but powerful message from my neck to "Stop working so hard and just love me!" It stopped me in my tracks! I realized I had separated from my neck and was "working" on "it." When I began to send love instead, my movements and my heart began to soften as did the pain and stiffness in my neck. I still do range of motion exercise for my neck, but now it is a soft and flowing dance rather than forcing my head to tilt and turn.

It is so important to learn what works best for your own body. The only constants are loving-kindness and an ability to listen to what your body is telling you. As you follow the experiences in each chapter you will get better and better at doing this.

Being Present

Self-massage can help you to become comfortable with your own company, to be present with yourself. When you are alone do you have a sense of feeling at home with yourself? Many people don't, but this sense of peace with ourselves is vital to expanding our sense of wholeness and well-being. If you are not at home with yourself, you cannot really be at home anywhere. This may feel like a difficult place to start, since so many people are not comfortable being alone without the television or computer or radio as a distraction. In fact, it may seem to you to be the most uncomfortable place to be. The good news is that listening to your body's messages and then giving kind touch to yourself leads in a simple way to feeling this sense of comfort with yourself. As you do this, you will begin to soften into your own wholeness. This kindness will expand to fill all of you—your body, mind, heart, and soul. Taking the time to develop a loving relationship with yourself brings the gift of completeness and knowing you are okay and can take care of your own needs.

Paying attention when you move is a simple way to begin to be present in your body also. The next time you walk anywhere (yes anywhere) notice where in your body you feel relaxed, where there is smooth movement, and where there are hitches or discomforts. Notice what your mind says about these messages so that you learn how you were taught to treat yourself when your body felt certain things. If you were taught to ignore pain so you could keep getting the job done, it may seem self-indulgent to take the time to pay attention to your discomforts. Learning to

notice subtle messages while moving not only helps you be more present in the moment, it also brings you more grace and enjoyment of movement. You could get up right now and experiment with this. Walk slowly enough to notice the subtleties, then fast enough to allow your arms to swing.

Expanding Your Experience of Wholeness

In our culture we've been encouraged to separate our experience of our bodies and souls, our minds and hearts, our bodies and minds. It's not easy to feel our wholeness; being in touch with our bodies, hearts, minds, and souls at the same time offers a great challenge. Bringing them all back together is soul work; it takes conscious focus to move toward that union. Some spiritual practices invite us to leave our bodies behind in our spiritual quest, or to stop noticing them during meditation. Yoga intends to bring bodies and souls together, but in our bottom-line, productivity-oriented culture many people focus instead on getting the right amount of stretch or the perfect posture. Many religions encourage us to judge the body and its desires as bad. Believing that we follow our bodies *or* our souls splits us off from a valuable part of ourselves. Self-massage, in the context of soul work, brings us back to ourselves in a grounded way that actually increases our ability to hold the experience of wholeness and Spirit in our busy lives.

I used to believe that being whole meant that I would always feel light and happy—only good things. I have come to realize that wholeness is not complete if it does not also include the shadow or painful parts of ourselves. Most of us have uncomfortable parts of ourselves that we ignore, resent or split off from. Instead of distancing ourselves from those parts and wishing they would just go away, we can become an ally to them. We must bring these parts back into ourselves;

Movement is something we are rather than something we do. We are verbs, not nouns.

Emilie Conrad Da'oud

it's the only way to become whole. Self-massage helps us release self-judgements and shows us how to hold all of ourselves in gentle, kind hands: the parts we like as well as the parts we don't like, don't want, or that are painful.

Being in touch with our wholeness extends outward, as well. It reminds us of how we belong in the world, connecting to ourselves, to the people around us, to the earth, to all beings, and to Spirit, which holds the mystery of life.

Giving/Receiving

To expand your experience of wholeness you must learn to be both giver and receiver of love. Self-massage teaches you to learn about receiving the gifts you give yourself. You have access to feedback from what your hands and fingers feel as they massage, and also from the inner sensations in your muscles and tissues. Shifting your attention back and forth between giving and receiving allows the massage to be guided by your body's responses. Tuning in to both muscles and hands at the same time brings more of a sense of wholeness and flow to the experience.

Balancing

Wholeness grows when we feel a sense of balance in our bodies and in our lives. Balance is a path, not a steady state. Our bodies are constantly adapting to the changes in the environment around us, to what we put into them (food, drink), and to what we ask of them (work, exercise), or don't ask of them. The first step in moving toward balance is noticing imbalances in our bodies (pain, stiffness, discomfort), hearts (sadness, anger), and minds (preoccupations, rationalizations, judgments). The question is when will we notice. When will we choose to act to bring ourselves back into balance? Will we respond right away? Or will we wait until the distress becomes too large to ignore and limits our

ability to function normally? If we wait, we then often blame ourselves for doing something wrong, compounding the imbalance with self-judgment. Rather than beating ourselves up for not staying in perfect balance, we will greatly enhance our effectiveness by learning to pay attention and responding appropriately to the continually shifting balance between doing and being, giving and receiving, the physical and the spiritual, work and play.

Loving, Forgiving

Coming to the point of loving our bodies usually involves forgiveness. We must forgive our bodies for not living up to our (unattainable) goals. Most of us think we are too thin or too fat, too tall or too short, don't have large enough breasts or muscles, aren't beautiful or good looking enough—the list goes on and on. We must release ourselves from self-criticism to learn what is best for each of our unique bodies. Treating yourself kindly will bring life to your body; you will look better because of what shines from your face and because your body moves with more grace.

Self-Blessing, the first exercise at the end of this chapter and on the KindTouch CD, gives a process of connecting with yourself in a conscious and kind way, bringing your awareness to who you are at your center. It focuses your attention through your hands, bringing the best of your heart, soul, and mind to your body. It brings comfort, happiness, and a sense of your connection with Spirit. Listening to this blessing helps me soften and feel whole. This exercise sets the stage for all the other exercises in the book. You can stop reading and do it now or wait until the end of the chapter.

Supporting Healing

Healing means to become whole. I understand this from a personal viewpoint. I feel healthy even though I have chronic condi-

In avoiding all pain and seeking comfort at all cost, we may be left without intimacy or compassion; in rejecting change and risk we often cheat ourselves of the quest; in denying our suffering we may never know our strength or our greatness.

Rachel Naomi Remen

tions and problems. In the traditional definition of health as the absence of illness I'd be excluded from the state of health; and I am not willing to be excluded. The biggest difference between my status and the traditional definition of health is that I cannot afford to take my body for granted. I cannot disregard it or its needs without paying the price of pain and fatigue. But really, can anyone?

Choosing Wholeness

When we are injured or ill we have an important choice to make. We can choose to ignore or resent the problem, in which case we split off from that part of ourselves and become fragmented. We can choose instead a path of acceptance and compassion that brings us closer to wholeness and the experience of well-being.

Self-massage is a powerful path to support healing. It helps us listen to what our bodies need. It gives us a means of treating ourselves kindly and compassionately every day, whether we are ill, injured, or well. We need daily experiences of our wholeness. Massage stimulates the endorphins that give us a sense of well-being as well as natural pain relief. It brings us the relaxation that slows racing hearts, lowers blood pressure, and calms our breathing. When we give ourselves kind touch every day, it can transform our relationship to ourselves from judgmental or depressed to accepting and loving. The body can become a powerful route to change the emotional and mental habits that come from treating ourselves poorly. "Ninety percent of our thoughts about ourselves are negative," says Alice Domar, Ph.D., director of the Mind/Body Center for Women's Health at Harvard Medical School.* I can more easily break out of negative thoughts about myself through kindness to my body than by just

telling myself to change those thoughts. Focusing on my body distracts me from those thoughts. After I give and receive the kindness of my own touch, I can use the kindness that has settled in my body to shift my thinking and feelings into self-acceptance and compassion.

You can have an experience of seeing the difference that comes when you give yourself kind touch in the second exercise at the end of this chapter.

Reclaiming Wholeness

If you don't heed the messages from your body when they are mild discomforts, the symptoms will grow as large as they need to be to get your attention. The more willing you are to hear your body's messages, the sooner you'll notice a symptom when it is small and more manageable. Many young people can get away with ignoring their bodies without immediate consequences. But I see many of these people later, coming for massage therapy to help with new problems at the site of an old injury they ignored.

If you have old injuries or illness that you didn't care for well, which now make you susceptible to problems or re-injury, or if you ignore or reject a particular part of your body, you can choose now to reclaim your wholeness by bringing that area back into yourself. The exercises in Chapter 12 will help you find your own way to a kind relationship with areas of difficulty.

Staying Whole

Once we learn how to move toward wholeness, we can use these abilities at the beginning of a new challenge, whether it is an illness, an injury, or a loss. Again, choice makes the difference. If in our first reaction we choose to distance ourselves from the prob-

---

*Quoted in *Ladies' Home Journal,* Feb., 2001. See her book, *Self-Nurture: Learning to Care for Yourself As Effectively As You Care for Everyone Else.*

Anna's Story

Before the surgery and then in the recovery room after the hysterectomy I was unthinkingly wincing with frustration, sometimes anger, and almost cursing whenever I would feel a cramping in my colon. I was working against myself, and then I remembered the *Self-Blessing* that you taught me. I thought to join self-massage and a compassionate, mothering attitude. I lay on my back in the hospital bed with my hands cupping and rubbing my stomach very gently. The power in the "simple" act of holding my tummy and rubbing it as if it were an injured, frightened child was astounding to me. There was an immediate calming of pain and of everything jarred and jagged. I believe the self-massage aspect of my recovery multiplied the potency of the meditative one several fold. It took only two days of this multi-leveled kind of mothering for the colon pains to fade into nothing. What hasn't faded is my feeling that something humbly miraculous happened, and can happen again. I am so thankful.

lem, we learn to notice that process sooner and can begin to choose healing approaches earlier. The goal is to move toward healing as the first impulse. With practice we can keep decreasing the time between the challenge and the healing response. When our minds and emotions are confused, disappointed, or angry at a new diagnosis or problem, going to our bodies returns us to ourselves. Simply placing a hand over your heart or stroking your chest can ground you, and remind you that you are greater than the current problem. It can give you access to your soul, the part of yourself that is beyond physical limitations, and connects you to Spirit. Then you can use these extraordinary resources to receive love and compassion, and to gain a greater perspective.

Embodying Spirit

We are beings created with both physical body and soul. We are not one or the other; we are inextricably joined together as mortal and Spirit, sacred and mundane. We need to learn how to hold both of these parts of ourselves as one to experience our wholeness.

Expanding Your Experience of Spirit

Developing a daily practice of kind touch, bringing the best of our hearts, minds, and souls to our bodies, and then receiving the gifts the body returns, gives us a means of experiencing Spirit in our bodies. There are many ways to do this. The simplest (and most difficult) is to focus our attention on our bodies, becoming aware of the miracle and mystery of form and function that works so well for us.

Grounding Spirit

Self-massage, connecting with our bodies in a kind and loving way, provides a powerful tool for experiencing our entirety and our connection with Spirit even in the midst of

our busy days. It reminds us of how we belong in the world, of our connection not only to ourselves and to Spirit, but to the earth and to all beings. The last exercise in this book asks you to review which of the experiences you most loved, and to make a plan of how to incorporate them into your life. It doesn't have to take a lot of time. Simply adding your full presence while you briefly rub an achy neck (while sitting at your desk thinking about a thorny issue) reminds you that you are more than the worker with a problem to solve. There are many ways to bring compassion to yourself in the course of a busy day that take only a few minutes, but increase focus and perspective to your life as well as love and enjoyment.

Summary

Self-massage gives us a way to learn about our own bodies from the inside. We can listen to how each muscle responds to different kinds of touch and learn what strokes help it soften. Memories and emotions get stored in our bodies, and as we give kind attention to each part of our bodies, we can begin to accept and then release the thoughts and feelings that arise.

Self-massage offers a concrete way of expanding awareness of our wholeness. It helps us release judgments about our bodies and ourselves, and to accept ourselves in the moment. We can move from judgment to gratitude when we focus our attention on our wholeness—body, mind, heart, and soul. From this perspective we then experience our connection with Spirit and truly know how and where we belong in this world. Self-massage connects us with the center of our beings, with our souls, and gives us a grounded sense of Spirit and the mystery of life.

SELF-BLESSING

Exercise 2a

Introduction

The *Self-Blessing* exercise—the first one on the *KindTouch CD*—guides you through a method of opening deeply to yourself. I recommend you do it in the morning and before you go to sleep at night. It creates a habit of self-kindness, greeting the divine in yourself, and reminding you of who you really are. After you become very familiar with this process, you can create your own personalized blessing to do each day. The script may be found in Appendix A at the end of the book.

You can do this in any position: sitting, standing, or reclining. You can do this blessing by physically following the steps, or you can be still physically and use the strong power of your imagination and inner sensations to experience the effects. For those of you with a meditation or imagery practice, it may be a more powerful experience to be still physically; the doing can be distracting from the inner experience. I recommend that everyone try this both ways; after a while of doing it physically, try resting your body and following the steps in your imagination.

Preparation

The first step is to create a comfortable environment for yourself. If something particular helps you feel relaxed, bring that into your space. You may like soft music or prefer it quiet. If you have any objects that evoke sacred space for you bring them in also. Wear loose clothing that doesn't bind, and gather a journal and favorite pen for recording your discoveries. Eliminate distractions like the phone. Do whatever helps you know you are entering a time to give yourself kind, focused attention. Then settle into the place you created for yourself.

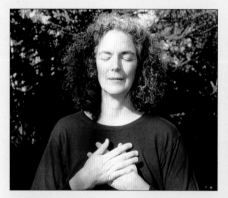
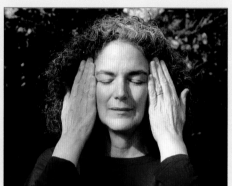
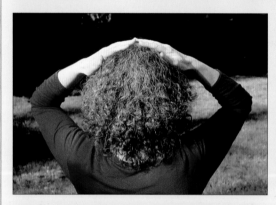
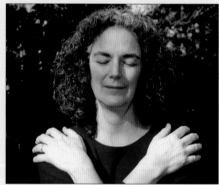
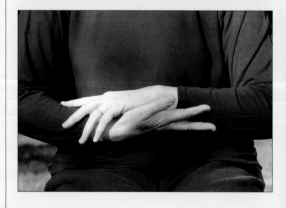
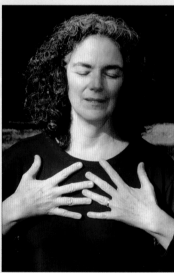

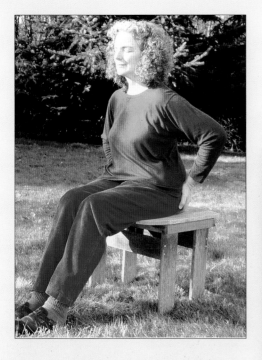

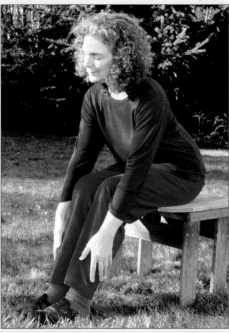

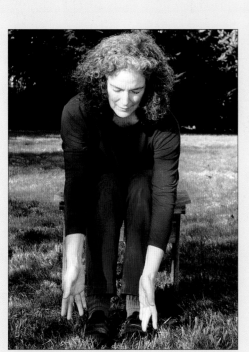

DIRECTIONS

1. Set aside fifteen to twenty minutes during which you won't be interrupted. Remove your glasses before beginning.
2. Listen to *Self-Blessing* on the *KindTouch CD.* Note that the exercise begins with taking eight slow breaths. You can take more than that if you need to; do whatever is relaxing for you.

Journal

Write about your experiences.

- How do you feel after doing this *Self-Blessing?*
- How fully were you able to become present for yourself?
- How would you describe the touch you gave yourself?
- Make a plan for when you will listen to this *Self-Blessing,* and visualize that in your daily schedule.

This Week

- Listen to *Self-Blessing* on the *KindTouch CD* every day. Try doing it in the morning and evening.
- Notice any ways you want to modify this *Self-Blessing* to personalize it for yourself.
- If you want, you can tape the blessing in your own voice with the changes you have made for yourself. (See Appendix A for the script.)

SEEING SOFTNESS
MIRROR EXERCISE #1

Exercise 2b

Introduction

Do this exercise at a separate time from the first one, since it also uses the *Self-Blessing*.

Most of us are used to looking at the surface appearance of our faces, and react to looking in the mirror in habitual ways. This exercise is an experience designed to bring your own typical responses to seeing your face into your consciousness, and then to see if and how that changes after spending some time using KindTouch.

Preparation

Gather your journal, pen, hand mirror, and anything you want to create a sacred space, and settle into your favorite spot.

DIRECTIONS

1. **Begin by looking at your face in the mirror for a few minutes and write down each thought and feeling as they arise, without censoring or judging them.**
2. **Listen to *Self-Blessing* on the KindTouch CD.**
3. **Afterwards, again look into the mirror at your face for a few minutes and record each of your thoughts and feelings.**
4. **Compare the two lists, and note down any differences before and after the *Self-Blessing*.**

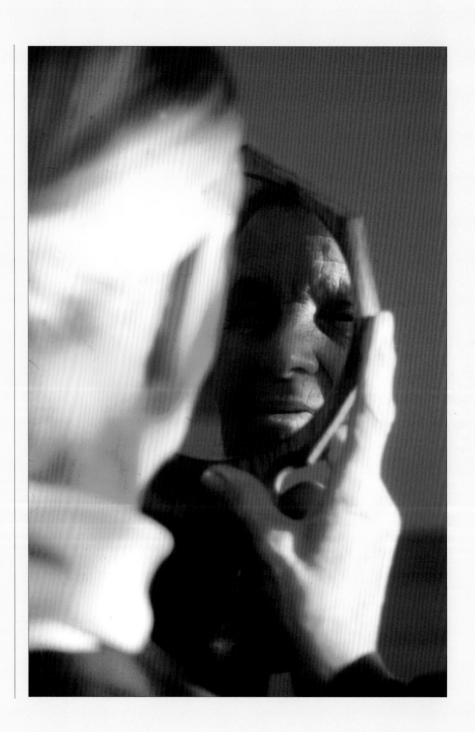

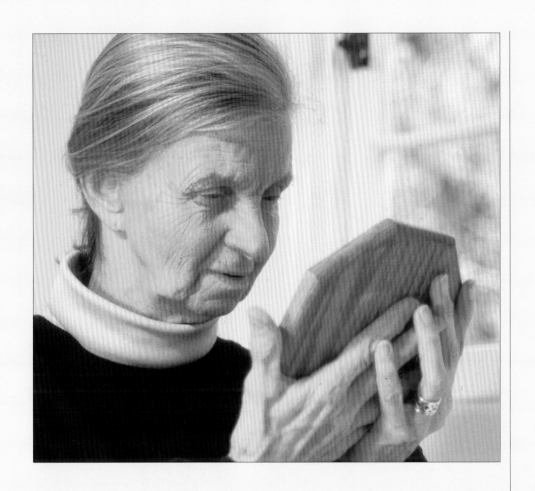

Journal

Write about your experiences

- Did you notice different kinds of things before and after the *Self-Blessing*?
- Were your feelings softer or more accepting?
- Why do you think your responses were similar or different?
- What qualities were easier to see after doing the *Self-Blessing*?

This Week

- Do the *Self-Blessing* on the *KindTouch CD* once or twice a day, noticing if and how it changes your experience of yourself and how your day goes. Note this in your journal.
- Consciously stretch your whole body at least once a day. Try stretching as a transition between activities or projects, especially if you spend long periods of time sitting at a desk.
- Once a day bring your awareness to how your body feels as you walk. Does the movement feel easy and flowing, or is there stiffness, or lack of ease? If you feel stiffness, slow down your movements and try different ways of moving your hips, your shoulders, your arms and legs. Moving slowly may allow your body to discover ways to feel more flowing and comfortable.

Chapter 3

Our Healing Spiral

he process of consciously healing ourselves moves us deeper into our experience of being whole. Health means the full experience of wholeness, which can take a lifetime to grow into. It takes congruity among all parts of ourselves—body, mind, heart, and soul. Congruence means agreement, harmony, or correspondence. The development of this congruence within ourselves creates a powerful healing state.

This view differs from the typical Western idea of health and illness as opposites, with cure or failure as the only outcomes. We need a larger container than cure or failure to hold the truth about health and illness, living and dying. If we only think of ourselves as healthy when everything is going right in our bodies, we will miss out on a lot of time that we could be feeling whole and good about ourselves in spite of an injury or illness or emotional pain. Health as wholeness can exist no matter what is happening in the body, whether vibrant and full of energy, sick and filled with pain, or even dying. Perhaps wholeness can especially be accessible when dying. The time before death can expand the experience of connection and wholeness even for people who have never known anything like it before.

Life as a Healing Journey

Each of us has a unique path that unfolds as we move through our lives. At different times we encounter love, pain, illness, healing, loss, peace, injury, growth, and untimately death. We tend to value and enjoy love, connection, and peace; and we devalue pain, fear, and separation. Yet with hindsight we often see that growth emerges from times of illness or emotional pain. These difficult experiences often become catalysts that enable us to allow more love and connection in our lives.

Our lives naturally flow back and forth between comfort and discomfort, in our bodies and in our emotions. Life in physical form means we are vulnerable through our bodies to pain and restriction as well as to pleasure and joy. Perhaps the most remarkable ability of the body is its power to heal itself.

Most of us can think of someone who has gone through a very difficult time in his or her life, perhaps a huge loss or a life-threatening illness or injury, and has emerged transformed. Facing this kind of trauma can help a person realize what is really important in life, and release what is not meaningful. Such a release comes only after great thought, emotion, and soul searching, and may result in a clarity and calmness that attracts others to learn more about them.

We are all already whole, but we rarely experience it or have the perspective to see it. This book is designed to give you experiences that will increase your ability to contact your inner wholeness. If you do the exercises you will learn to open more to each part of yourself—body, mind, heart, and soul.

The **body** is the physical vessel that we live in, our mortal aspect that exists along with the sacred in us. Our bodies have great wisdom that can teach us vital lessons about all aspects of ourselves. Physical symptoms are messengers about our next step in growth, and can become great allies rather than burdens. The **mind** also has great power in our lives. It brings reason and knowledge (the left or linear brain), creativity and intuition (the right or intuitive brain). The mind can provide vast gifts and also can interfere with our inner peace, if we get too caught up in its convolutions. The **heart** holds our emotions and gives us the capacity to love and to express our caring and compassion. It leads us to the things that are most deeply fulfilling, and connects us with our specific talents and gifts. It brings us to close connections with family, friends, and the world, and is the window to our soul. **Soul** is the divine spark in us, the deepest and largest part of us, always connected to Spirit. The soul holds the voice of inner wisdom and unconditional love for ourselves and others.

Most people have come to prefer certain of life's experiences and deny and reject others, unaware of the value of the hidden things that may come wrapped in plain or even ugly paper.

Rachel Naomi Remen

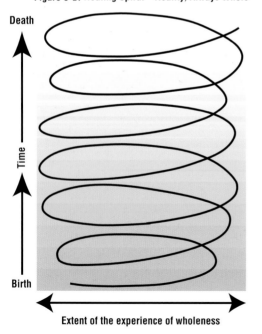

Figure 3-A: Healing Spiral – Ideal life

Death

Time

Birth

Extent of the experience of wholeness

Figure 3-B: Healing Spiral – Reality, Always Whole

Death

Time

Birth

Extent of the experience of wholeness

As our highest self or higher consciousness, it is the only part of us that is large enough to hold all of our joy and sadness, love and disappointment, ease and pain. Our bodies, minds, and hearts cannot quite wrap themselves around all the positive and negative experiences that exist side by side in us. Things that confuse our minds, pain our bodies, or sadden our hearts can always be held in compassion and wholeness in our souls.

In our society, we see health and disease as opposites, and we all know which is "good" and which is "bad." A person is "healthy" if they are disease-free today, but if they are diagnosed with cancer or diabetes tomorrow they have "lost their health." They are still the same person with the same condition; the only thing that has changed is that they received a diagnosis. In fact, it may turn out that the diagnosis leads them to actions that increase their health, to treatments and decisions that can improve their condition, or to discoveries that reconnect them to what is important in their lives. This holds true for emotional issues also. Depression and anxiety are widespread in our culture, and they are seen and treated as disease. What if we examined this trend to search for the underlying message it may convey about our priorities as a social system? Do we really want to suggest that a person with a chronic illness or irreparable disability must be defined as unhealthy throughout his or her life? What if we look at health and illness in terms of wholeness? Does this make a difference in our view of the quality of our lives?

Each of us has a powerful choice in how we respond to illness or pain. We can distance ourselves from the problem, or we can choose to move toward the difficulty, and thus toward wholeness. We can see the illness as a loss of health, or we can deepen our understanding of the illness and find a way to care for ourselves and remain whole. There is potential for growth in illness or pain or any

physical restriction, if we only know how to open to it and find it.

Symptoms are messengers. They can tell us that we must re-examine our priorities; that we demand too much from ourselves, or that we need more time alone or with family or friends, more rest, more play, more challenge. The message will be unique for each person and each situation. Learning its meaning offers a powerful avenue for deepening our connectedness with life and the impetus to give ourselves what we need.

The Healing Spiral

Rather than seeing love, contentment, vitality, connection, and absence-of-disease as the only positive ways to be, and running from pain and displeasure, we can see life as a spiral, a life-long healing journey, where we move through both smooth and difficult times. This spiral holds all of our experiences without judgment. The opposites of health versus illness, of contentment versus sorrow do not exist in the spiral. Each experience and feeling brings something of value to our lives and helps move us along our own healing spiral toward a greater sense of wholeness.

Typically, a straight line is used to illustrate health and illness, with "health" on the right end and "illness" and "death" on the left. There are no straight lines in the healing spiral, no right and left, only curves that always move forward through time. Since there is no judgment about good or bad, an experience enters into the spiral based on when it happens in time, not on a health-illness continuum. It doesn't matter if it lands on the right side, the front, the left, or the back of the spiral. The width of the spiral at any given time represents the degree to which a person is experiencing wholeness at that moment. Wider curves reflect times when the person is feeling a greater sense of wholeness, while narrow coils represent times when the person feels constricted and is less in touch with wholeness. Constrictions generally happen in response to a new life challenge, such as an illness, injury, loss or other difficulty. It also can happen when a person enters any new life experience; a new job, new marriage, new school, new move, new baby. Each of us has a unique path through our own spiral that reflects our life experiences and our inner ability to call upon our wholeness to respond to challenges.

You can use the spiral as a way to plot your life's journey, to help you identify your patterns of response, both to traumas and to smooth sailing. You can also use it to look at your typical fluctuations as you move through an average day. Do you generally wake up feeling good and whole, overwhelmed, looking forward to your day, or resisting what you must do? How does your day tend to evolve, in terms of when you expand and when you contract?

The first illustration of a spiral (Figure 3-A) shows the overview of a life thats grows and deepens into an ever-increasing sense of wholeness from birth to death. No one's life follows this smooth path, but this example shows the outlines of an ideal progression toward complete awareness of ourselves as whole. The reality is that we are always whole even though we may not be in touch with that reality all the time. (See Figure 3-B.)

Figure 3-C gives an example of a more realistic lifetime spiral, with its ups and downs, ins and outs, times of a full sense of wholeness and then times of trauma when that wholeness feels threatened. It shows the typical constriction after a shock and then the working back to wholeness. Sometimes we come back to a smaller sense of wholeness, and sometimes to more, depending on how fully we incorporate the experience and deepen our sense of who we are.

The fourth illustration (Figure 3-D) shows a few occurrences over the course of one person's day, demonstrating their effects on her experience of wholeness. Of course, there is a myriad of experiences that happen moment to moment in anyone's day. Figure 3-D offers a simple example you can follow to track your own experience of wholeness throughout the day.

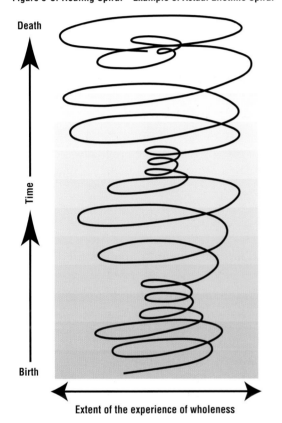

Figure 3-C: Healing Spiral – Example of Actual Lifetime Spiral

Death

Time

Birth

Extent of the experience of wholeness

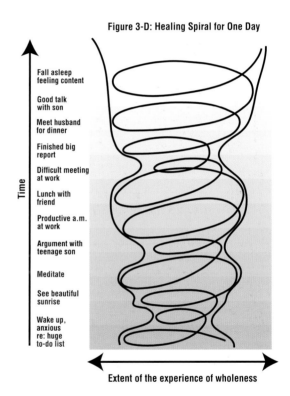

Figure 3-D: Healing Spiral for One Day

Time

Fall asleep feeling content

Good talk with son

Meet husband for dinner

Finished big report

Difficult meeting at work

Lunch with friend

Productive a.m. at work

Argument with teenage son

Meditate

See beautiful sunrise

Wake up, anxious re: huge to-do list

Extent of the experience of wholeness

THE MEANING OF HEALING AND WHOLENESS

Exercise 3a

Preparation

Settle into a comfortable position in the area you've prepared for yourself and begin to turn your focus inward, allowing your eyes to close or to have a soft downward gaze.

Take eight slow, deep breaths, using them to bring yourself fully present. Use the first two to replace tension in your body with softness throughout. With the next two breaths allow your mind to quiet and focus only on being present right now. Let the next two breaths open your heart; feel the warm light of the love in your heart filling your whole being. With the next two breaths expand your awareness of your soul and your connection with Spirit, sensing the wisdom, love, and healing within and around you.

Let yourself feel grounded as if you had roots that extend down into the nourishing soil. With a sense of peace and comfort, begin the exercise.

DIRECTIONS

1. **Take a few minutes to write about your own definitions of healing, health, and wholeness.**
   - **Have your ideas changed after giving yourself kind attention and touch in the *Self-Blessing* and after reading this chapter regarding beliefs about healing?**
   - **Do you believe an illness, injury or loss can bring you to greater wholeness? How? Or why not?**

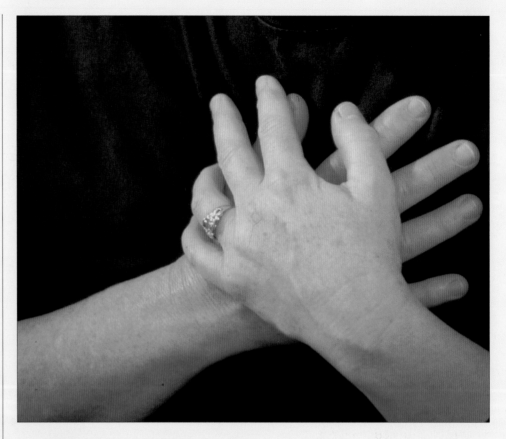

- **Have you had an experience with injury, illness, or loss?**
- **If so, what did you learn, and how did you deepen your sense of wholeness as a result of the trauma?**
- **Where do you feel you are in your life now on your healing path?**

This Week

- Let your mind, heart, body, and soul revisit your sense about healing during this week.
- Talk with family or friends about your ideas.
- Note your insights in your journal.

HEALING SPIRAL
FOR A DAY

Exercise 3b

Preparation

Settle into a comfortable position in the area you've prepared for yourself and begin to turn your focus inward, allowing your eyes to close or to have a soft downward gaze.

Take eight slow, deep breaths, using them to bring yourself fully present. Use the first two to replace tension in your body with softness throughout. With the next two breaths allow your mind to quiet and focus only on being present right now. Let the next two breaths open your heart; feel the warm light of the love in your heart filling your whole being. With the next two breaths expand your awareness of your soul and your connection with Spirit, sensing the wisdom, love, and healing within and around you.

Let yourself feel grounded as if you had roots that extend down into the nourishing soil. With a sense of peace and comfort, begin the exercise.

DIRECTIONS

1. **Draw your own spiral to see what (or when) causes a constriction in the experience of your wholeness.**
   - **List the events in chronological order on the left, starting at the bottom.**
   - **Then add your spiral, illustrating expansions and contractions in your experience of wholeness.**
2. **Where in your body do you feel the constriction?**
3. **What helps you to fully expand into your wholeness?**
4. **Take a moment to bring your kind touch to this area, and note in your journal what happens when you do.**

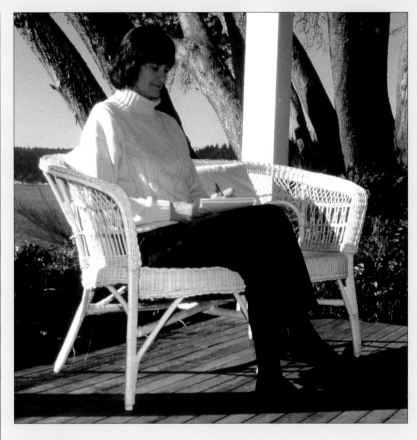

This Week

- Whenever you feel yourself constricting, notice where you feel it in your body. Take a minute (or ten) to touch that area kindly, to remind yourself of your wholeness.
- Continue doing the *Self-Blessing* once or twice every day. Write about any shifts you notice in your experience.
- For several days, pay attention to the constriction and expansion that you experience. Do you notice a pattern? Do you often wake up constricted, or feeling open and whole? What about when you go to work, or come home, or go to bed?
- If you would like, create a similar healing spiral for your whole life.

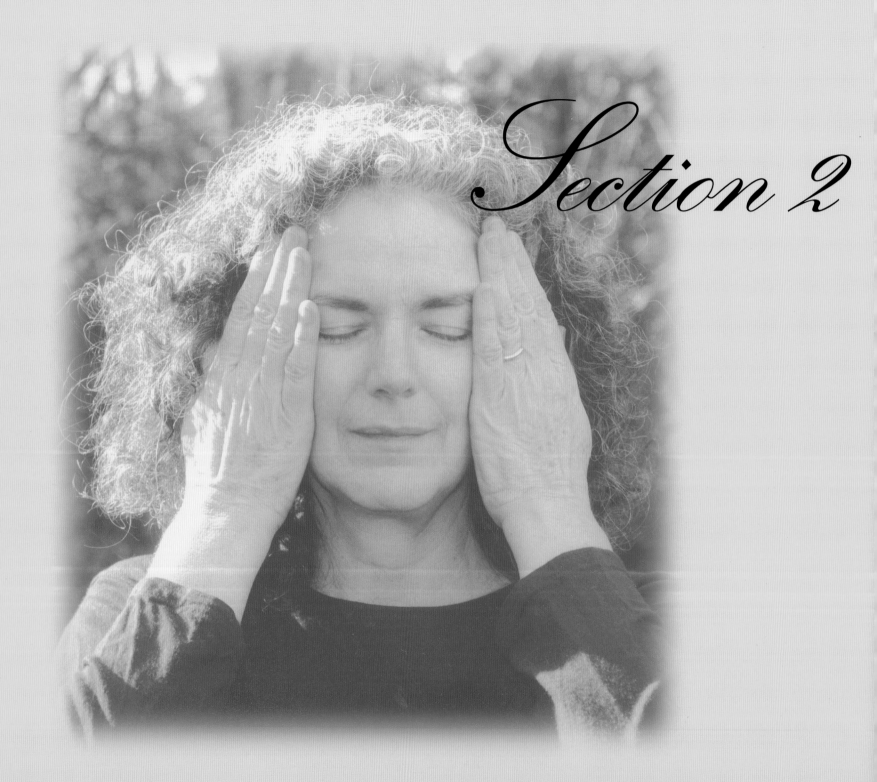

Section 2

Learning the Language of Touch

Touching is the oldest language, and kind touch is magic. Touch conveys subtleties of emotion and thought, and it brings comfort and relaxation. It is even more important to learn this language today, since in our culture we do little touching except with lovers and small children. We can reclaim our own role in our healing path when we give ourselves kind touch. It can open the door to deeper comfort and healing than we have ever experienced before. We often believe our own touch is less valuable than having someone else massage us, but we don't arrange to have massages, and end up going without. When we always look to others to give us comfort and love, we ignore the most important sources: ourselves, and Spirit within us.

Your body will tell you where and how it wants to be touched if you listen well. The first step in learning what your body wants and needs in self-massage is to learn the language of kind touch. This is the language through which you will communicate with your body. This section will teach you some of the basic strokes of massage therapy, adapted for self-massage. You already know much of what you need. The purpose is not that you will learn a certain formula for applying techniques to your body. Instead I hope you will learn the strokes simply as a vocabulary of touch so that you will feel comfortable in approaching each part of your body in several ways. Approach each stroke with curiosity and openness so you can absorb not only the how-to directions but also the purpose and spirit of the movement.

As with any new skill, you need to learn the tools first. In Chapters 4-8 you will learn how to apply each stroke to different areas of your body: your face and head, neck and shoulders, arms and hands, torso, legs and feet. After you have practiced and feel you are getting comfortable with the movements, Chapter 9 will lead you through a pictorial overview of a complete self-massage for relaxation, combining all the strokes as you move through your body. There is also a guided half-hour relaxation massage on the *KindTouch CD* that you can follow. Once you learn how to combine the strokes and know what your body likes best, you can follow your own intuition to create a self massage unique to your needs.

Often hands will solve a mystery that the intellect has struggled with in vain.

C.G. Jung

Strokes

Each chapter covers one stroke, giving general instructions and including variations for each part of your body, moving from your head to your toes. Photographs demonstrate the different approaches you can try. Taking the time to practice each stroke for each part of your body as you read will give you a sense of how to do each one in a variety of areas. Large muscled areas need the whole hand to massage them, while smaller muscles may only need the tips of the fingers. Trust yourself as you experiment with these strokes. Try them gently and with more pressure, faster and slower, listening to the response in your muscles and learning what your body likes.

You will develop your own style, just as each massage therapist even from the same school ends up with his or her own unique style. The way you massage yourself will be just right for you when you listen well to your own body. Make notes in your journal as you experiment with the strokes in this section, writing down your preferences for pressure and style for each area of your body.

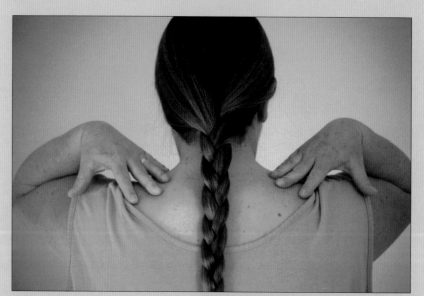

Gliding (effleurage)

In gliding, make long smooth strokes in the direction of the muscle fibers, molding your hands or fingers to the body contours. In general, heavier pressure goes toward the heart, lighter pressure can go either direction.

Kneading or squeezing (petrissage)

In kneading, conform your hands or fingers to the tissue and lift, squeeze, and knead it away from the underlying structure. You can use one or two hands, using the flats of your fingers, lifting them toward the heel of your hand or your flat thumb in a firm circular motion. Start at the area closest to the heart and gradually move down the limb or area you are working on. Always follow with a firm, gliding stroke toward your heart.

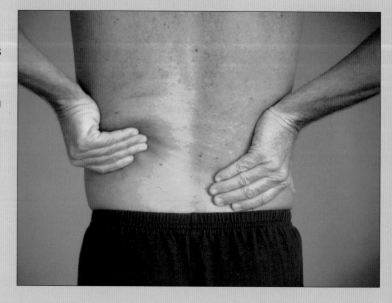

In addition to the five basic strokes pictured below and described in detail in the following chapters, I want to mention a stroke we often ignore: **holding,** attentively resting your hand on an uncomfortable area. There is great power in simply resting your hand(s) on a tight or painful spot if you bring your presence and kindness to that area as you hold it. The warmth of your hand brings a message to (and from) each part of yourself – body, mind, heart, and soul. When you "listen" to the tight area you may sense a shift in the uncomfortable sensation simply from bringing your kind attention to it. An easy place to experience this is to rest your hands on your abdomen when it is uncomfortable. This amount of physical warmth combined with an attentive and kind posture is surprisingly soothing to the organs in the abdomen. See Chapter 12 for more experience in holding with presence.

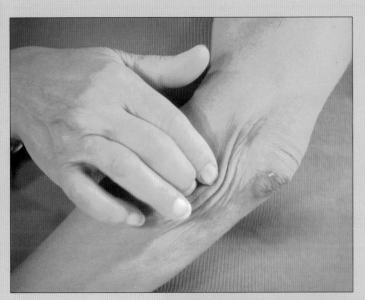

Friction

In friction strokes, compress the tissue with your fingers, thumbs or hands, moving the surface layers over the underlying structures. This is a more focused stroke than the others and generally moves across the direction of the muscle fibers. Always follow friction with gliding.

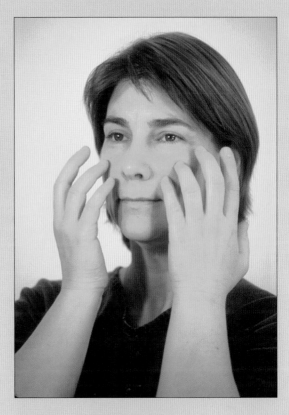

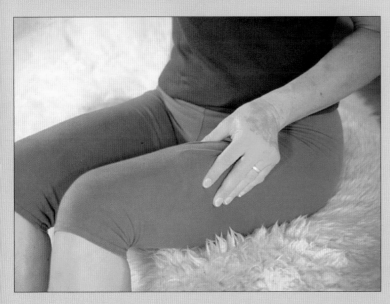

Vibration

One way to do vibration is to grasp the muscle and shake it back and forth.

Tapping (tapotement)

Tapping is done only over areas with bones under them, that is, not the low back or abdomen. Tapping is a percussive movement using very relaxed hands or fingers. On the face, it is done very lightly, using only the fingers. Otherwise, the movement is from the wrist and is light and smooth.

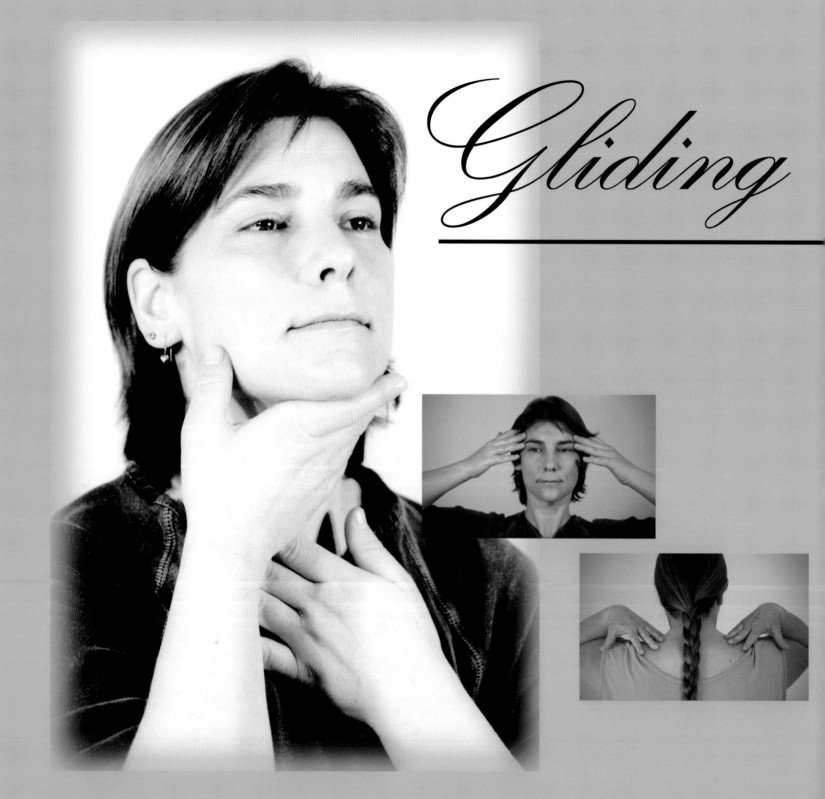

Gliding

Chapter 4 – Gliding

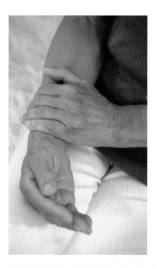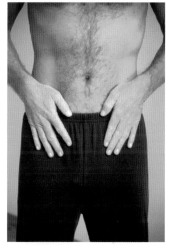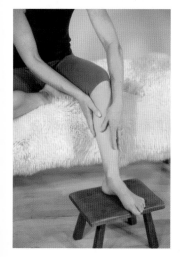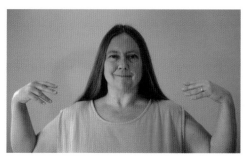

GLIDING or effleurage strokes are straight, smooth strokes. Molding your hand to the contours of your body, make the stroke in the direction of the muscle fibers. Depending on the size of the area you are massaging, you can use your whole hand, the side of your hand, the flats of your fingers, or for small areas the pads (not the tips) of the fingers.

Begin working in an area with lighter gliding strokes, using light pressure in long, smooth strokes. It is important to begin and end massage work this way. It gets the muscles used to being touched at the start, allows them to relax into the massage, and prepares them for a more focused touch. Without this preparation muscles may tighten against an unexpected deeper touch. At the end of a massage or between deeper strokes, gliding calms and completes the experience. When done lightly this stroke can go either direction, up or down a muscle.

If you are **using oil,** this stroke spreads the oil evenly. Spread the oil over the palms of your hands and apply it gradually as you glide over the area you are massaging. If you are wearing clothes, they can take the place of oil, allowing your hands to glide over the surface of your body. Thinner, more form-fitting clothes like tights help you to glide either up or down a muscle more easily without dealing with bunching clothes.

You can progress to using more pressure in the gliding strokes. With deeper pressure the movement needs to be directed toward the heart in order to protect the delicate valves in your veins and to direct waste products into the lymphatic system for removal. Heavier pressure with gliding helps your circulation by squeezing the blood through your veins and fluid through your lymph vessels toward your heart. It is very relaxing to tired and aching muscles. Improved circulation and lymph flow help remove waste products from fatigued, sore muscles. Better blood flow brings more nutrients and oxygen to the area to support the self-healing process that goes on all the time in our bodies. It also stimulates the parasympathetic nervous system, which gives a calming effect to the whole body as well as the mind and emotions.

Nerve strokes are a specialized type of gliding, using the fingertips to very gently stroke the skin away from the heart toward the tips of the fingers or toes. These are soothing, smoothing, and releasing strokes, and they have a relaxing and balancing effect on the nervous system. You can do these in one long stroke or in a series of shorter brushing strokes with the movement always progressing down the body. The fingertips barely touch the skin. It is nice to start the nerve strokes with shorter brushing strokes, and then follow up with a longer, slower stroke or two. You can feel the relaxation that flows down your body, calming you. If you are tuned in to your energy flow you can feel these strokes smooth, balance, and unruffle your energy and release blockages.

Deep-focused gliding will be covered under Chapter 6: Friction, as its purpose is to focus narrowly on a specific muscle rather than to glide over a broad area.

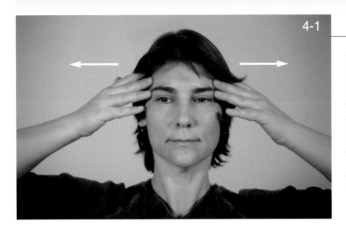

4-1: Stroke your fingers from the center of your forehead to your temples several times, experimenting with different amounts of pressure. Try this with the pads of your fingertips and with the flats of your fingers.

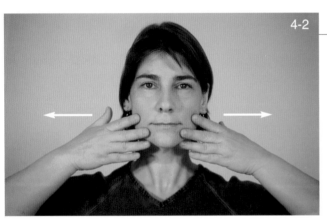

4-2: Stroke your fingers from your nose across your cheeks, and then across your lips and jaw. Experiment with different amounts of pressure.

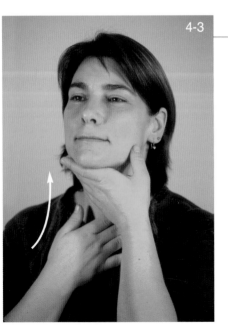

4-3: Stroke your fingers up your throat in a gentle glide, alternating hands. You can also use the backs of your fingers for this stroke.

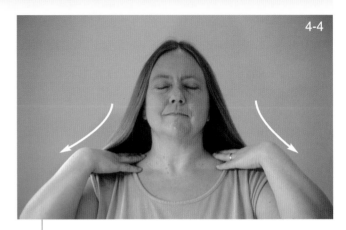

4-4: Glide your hands down the sides of your neck and across the tops of your shoulders several times. You can increase your pressure as you go if you want.

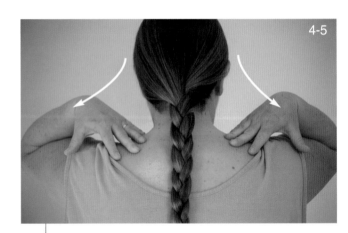

4-5: Glide down the back of your neck and across the tops and back of your shoulders. You can use more pressure here with these bigger, stronger muscles.

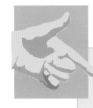

Remember that lighter strokes can go in both directions on muscles, and toward or away from the heart. Reserve deeper pressure for gliding strokes toward the heart.

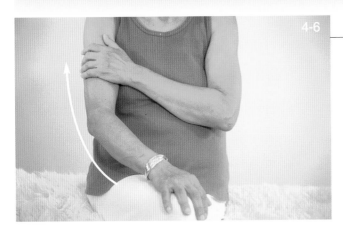

4-6: Glide your hand from wrist to shoulder, letting your hand conform to the shape of your arm as you go. Repeat for both sides of your arm. Let your hand glide gently back down to your starting point, and repeat with deeper pressure on the upward stroke.

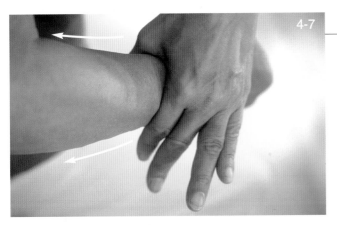

4-7: You can use more pressure for your forearm if you place your thumb on the inside of your arm and your fingers on the outer side.

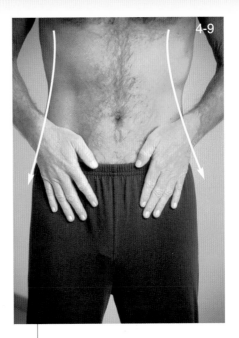

4-9: Glide the palms of your hands from your chest down over your abdomen and slide off the sides of your hips.

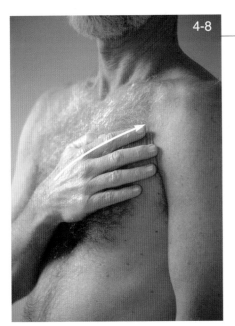

4-8: Glide the palm of your hand from the center of your chest outward to your arm just below your shoulder. Your "pecs" or pectoralis major muscle attaches to your arm there. Refer to photo 5-8 to see how this muscle forms the front of the axilla (arm pit).

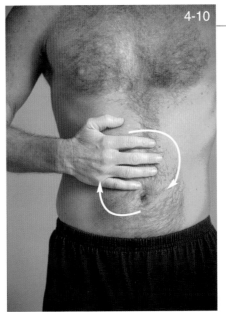

4-10: Hold your hand over your abdomen and bring your kind attention to any area of discomfort. Glide in a circle, making sure you move up the right side, across your upper abdomen, and down the left side so you go with your bowel, not against it. Make several slow circles.

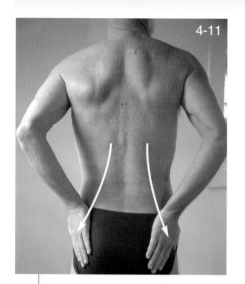

4-11: Begin as far up your back as is comfortable for you, and glide down and across your buttocks.

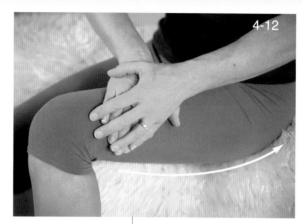

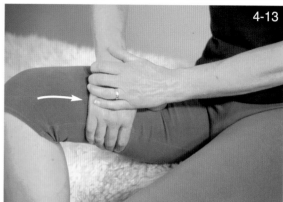

4-12 & 4-13: Placing one hand over the other to increase the amount of pressure for these large muscles, glide your hands up all four sides of your thigh, continuing up the side of your hip. Gently glide back down.

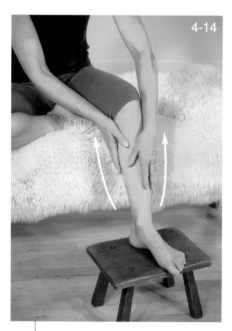

4-14: Glide up your lower leg from your ankle to your knee, either with one hand, or with both hands on opposite sides of your leg.

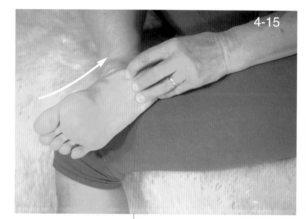

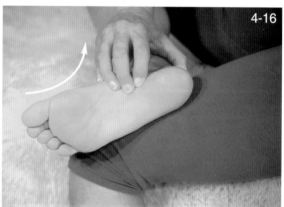

4-15 & 4-16: Glide the tips of your curved fingers from the ball of your foot to your heel, then again from the ball of your foot up across your arch, using as much pressure as your foot enjoys. Then glide your fingers up across the top of your foot.

N E R V E   S T R O K E S

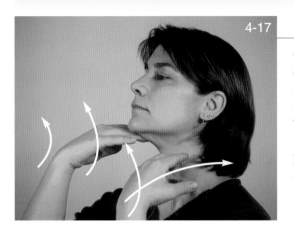

4-17: Glide over your whole face and neck, lightly touching your skin with the fingertips. Explore how stroking in different directions feels. You can extend these nerve strokes over and around your head or down your throat as you do in the *Self-Blessing* Exercise 2a.

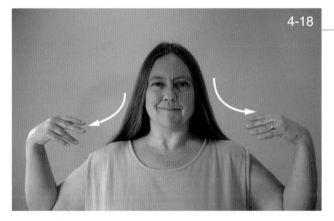

4-18: Draw your fingertips across the sides, back and front of your neck and shoulders.

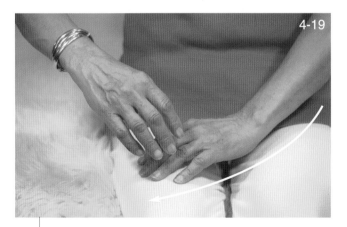

4-19: Slide your fingertips softly down your arms and hands, gliding off the ends of your fingers. You can use shorter brushing strokes at first and end with a longer soothing one.

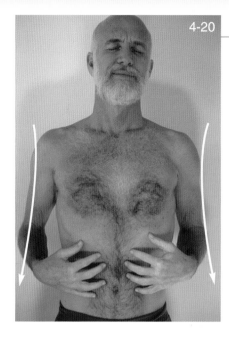

4-20: Gently glide down and across your chest and abdomen, sliding off the sides of your hips.

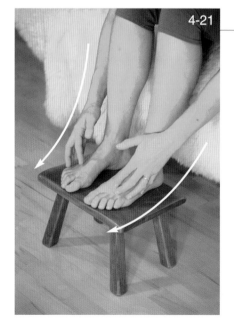

4-21: Softly glide your fingertips down your legs to your feet, and off your toes. Try brushing your fingertips down each leg, alternating hands, and end with a longer light stroke.

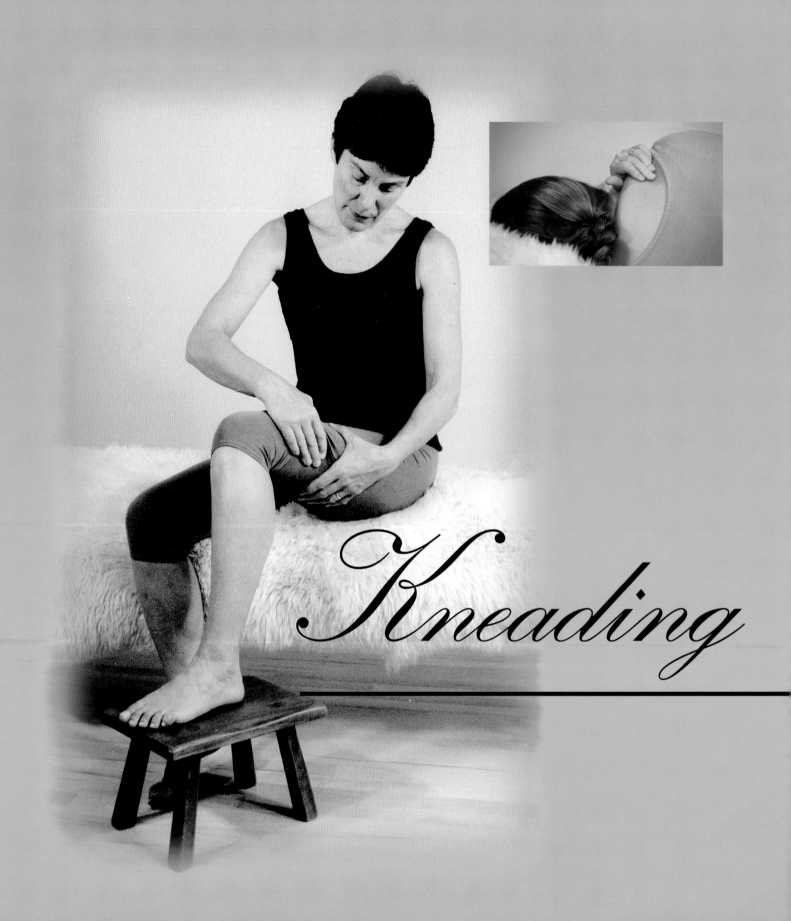

Kneading

Chapter 5 – *Kneading*

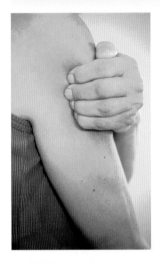

NEADING or petrissage is similar to kneading dough for bread, except that instead of pressing the dough down into the table, the direction of pressure is upward. You lift the muscles up and away from the underlying structures. In this stroke you let your hands conform to the shape of the muscle tissue you are working on, with your fingers on one side and either the heel of your hand or the flat surface of your thumb on the other side. Then use your fingers as a unit, lifting, squeezing, and kneading the tissue away from the underlying structure. Use a firm circular movement. It is good to begin at the end of the muscle that is closest to the heart and start each squeezing movement a bit farther down the muscle.

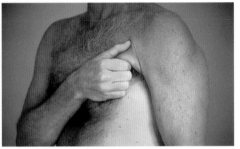

Always follow kneading with a gliding stroke toward the heart to relax the muscles and to move the waste products you have just mobilized into the circulatory and lymph systems. You can knead an area once or several times, gliding back up to the starting point each time.

Kneading helps prevent muscle stiffness after exertion by releasing waste products into the circulatory system and stimulating blood and lymph flow. Kneading stretches the tissue, reduces congestion, invigorates the skin, and relaxes the whole area.

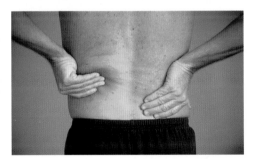

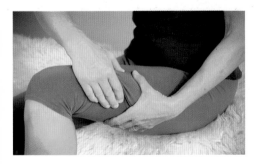

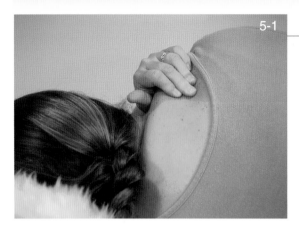

5-1

5-1: Knead each side of your neck and shoulder with the opposite hand so the muscles you are massaging aren't working and can relax. This can be done sitting up, or you can lie down so the muscles can really let go. Remember to lift the muscles away from the bones, with your fingers moving toward the heel of your hand. Imagine the effects spreading into your upper back. Continue kneading up the side of your neck.

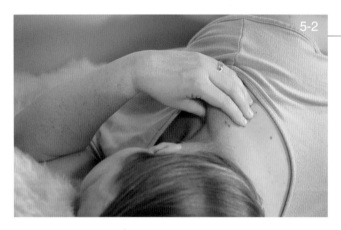

5-2

5-2: You can also knead your neck and shoulder by lifting your fingers toward the soft pad of your thumb. If you do this sitting up, rest your lower arm and hand in your lap or on the arm of your chair so that your shoulder muscles can rest. Continue kneading up the side of your neck.

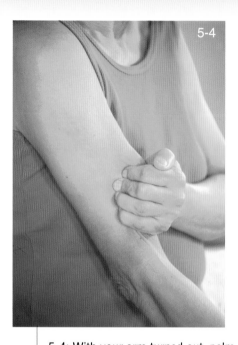

5-4

5-4: With your arm turned out, palm up, knead the bicep muscle in the front of your upper arm, lifting your fingers up toward the heel of your hand. Begin at your shoulder, moving down to your elbow. Then glide back up across your shoulder.

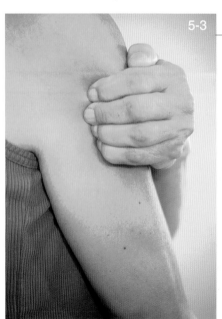

5-3

5-3: Knead your upper arm by pulling your fingers toward the heel of your palm with a lifting squeeze. Begin at the top of your arm, working around from the front to the back to massage the front, side, and back sections of the deltoid muscle.

5-5: Knead your tricep muscle in the back of your upper arm, beginning at the upper end, moving down to your elbow, and then gliding back up over your shoulder.

Remember to note your preferences in your journal.

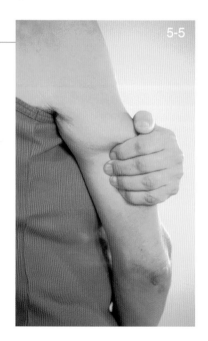

5-5

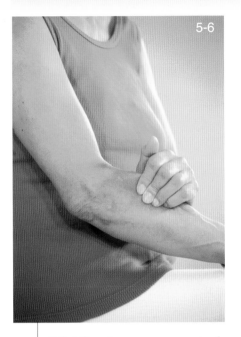

5-6: Lift and squeeze your outer forearm muscles, using your fingers against the heel of your hand. Begin at the elbow and move down, completing with a glide back up.

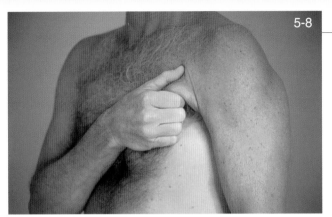

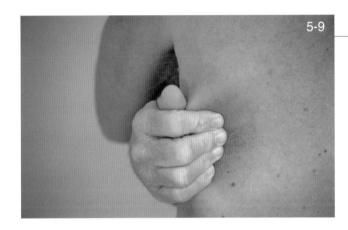

5-8: Grasp your "pec" muscle, (the pectoralis major) and lift your fingers toward the heel of your hand, moving from the tendon where it attaches to your arm over to your breast bone. Avoid breast tissue.

5-9: Knead the muscles over your ribs between your fingers and the heel of your hand, reaching around as far as comfortable to your side and back, and moving down and around your waist. In your imagination, feel the effects of this stroke spread across your back.

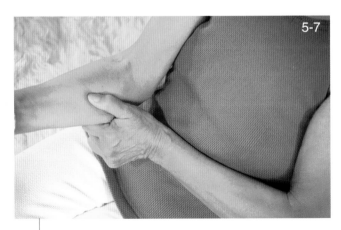

5-7: For the inner side of your forearm, turn your palm up and use your fingers against the flat length of your thumb, beginning at your elbow. Glide back up.

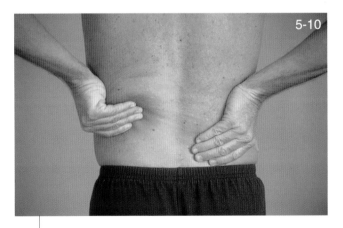

5-10: Place your hands only as far up your back as you are comfortable reaching, and alternate the action of your hands as you knead each side of your low back, pulling your fingers toward the heels of your hands.

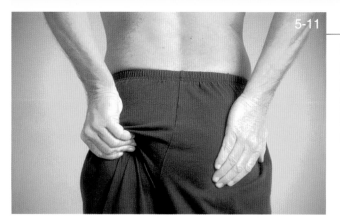

5-11: Knead the large, hard-working muscles of your buttocks by lifting your fingers toward the heels of your hands. Alternate hands with the strokes, gradually moving out to the sides.

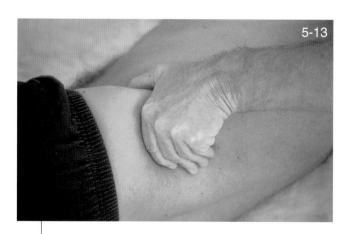

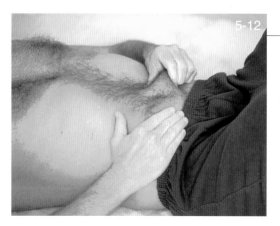

5-12: Lying down with your knees bent, knead your abdomen using both hands. Lift the surface tissues with your fingers against your flat thumbs, gradually covering your whole abdomen.

5-13: Lying on your side, knead the muscles on the side of your waist, lifting your fingers up to your flat thumb. You can walk your hand around from your back to the front.

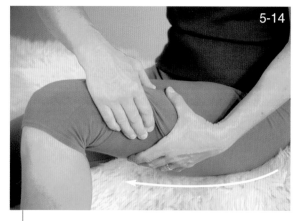

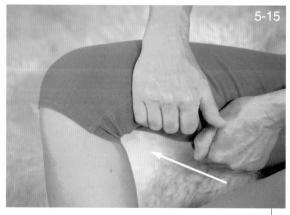

5-14 & 5-15: Use both hands to knead the large muscles in your legs. For the front and sides of your thigh, point your hands in the same direction. Alternately pull the fingers of one hand and then the other toward either the flat surface of your thumb or the heel of your hand. Try both; each may be easier with different sides of your leg. You can also push forward with one hand while the other pulls back. Practice until you feel an easy rhythm. Knead from your hip to your knee, and glide back up.

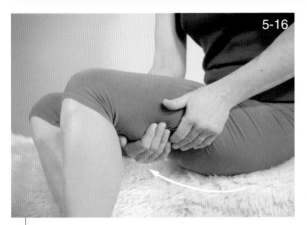

5-16

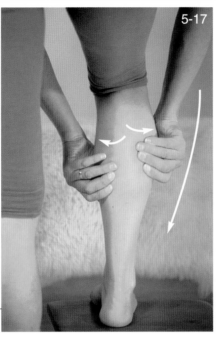

5-17

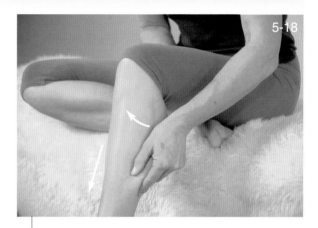

5-18

5-16 & 5-17: For the back of your leg, pull your fingers up toward the heel of each hand. You can continue down the whole leg and glide back up. It works easiest sitting with your foot resting on a stool.

5-18: The muscles on the front and outside of your lower leg are narrower and attached more closely to the bones, so they won't lift up as much. Knead with one hand, pulling your fingers toward your flat thumb. Move from knee to ankle, gliding back up.

Remember to note your preferences in your journal.

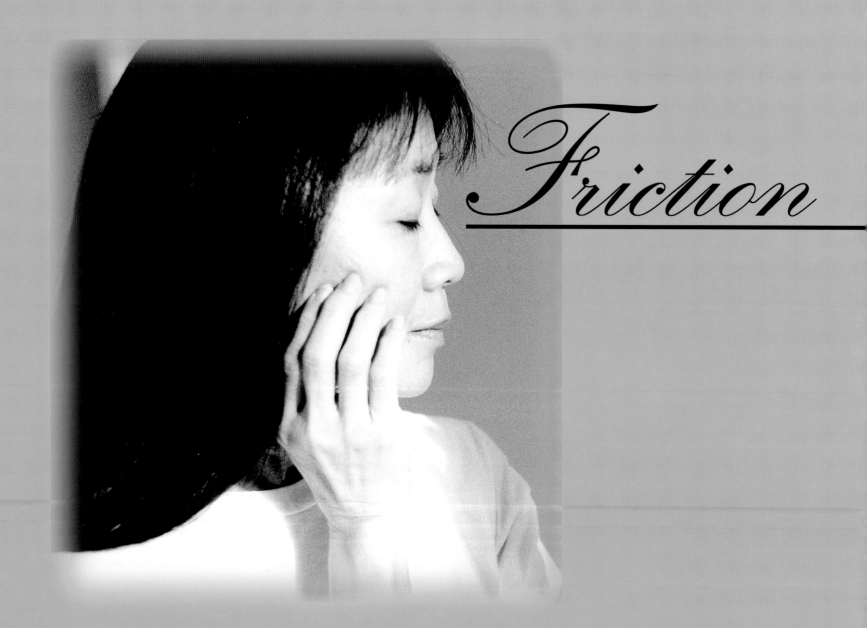

Friction

Chapter 6 - *Friction*

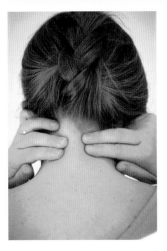

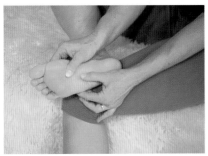

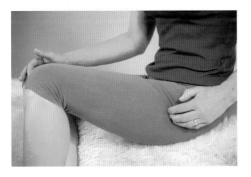

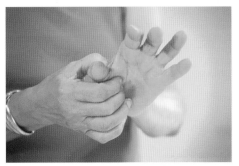

*R*UBBING or **FRICTION** is a way to focus more specifically in a painful or tight area. It requires sensitivity in your fingertips and that you stay in tune with the sensations in that tender spot. You can use variations of this stroke to stimulate and warm up large areas of the body. Friction also helps loosen scar tissue, such as adhesions or microscopic scarring that forms in the healing of any kind of injury; and it helps to release hypertonicities (too much muscle tone, making the muscle too tight) following exercise or chronic tension in an area. It stretches and separates muscle fibers, increasing flexibility and decreasing restrictions in movement. Rapid strokes warm up the skin and surface tissues, increasing circulation ("in with the good"–oxygen and nutrients; "out with the bad"–waste products). Friction strokes can also help decrease swelling in an area by compressing the tissues and squeezing fluid out toward the lymph and blood circulation. Be cautious with this stroke; do not use it for areas that are quite swollen.

The techniques of friction vary a bit, but all include compression of the tissue and moving the superficial layers over the underlying structures. The movement is faster than gliding or kneading. Friction strokes usually include both hands, so we must adapt them for use in self-massage, except for areas that both hands can reach: the legs and feet, the chest and abdomen. Movement is typically across the fibers of the muscles.

Cross-fiber friction involves moving your fingertips or thumbs across the direction the muscle fibers run. The amount of pressure is varied depending on how large or tender the muscles are. For example, gentle pressure is used for the face, while deeper pressure is used for the thighs.

Circular thumb or circular finger friction is a variation on cross-fiber friction, where the thumbs or fingers make alternating circles across the muscle fibers as they move along the length of a muscle.

Deep-focused gliding is technically not a friction stroke, but is included here because it concentrates on a small, focused area and uses deeper pressure as in the other friction strokes. The pressure is made with the fingertips or thumbs and follows the muscle and tendon from beginning to end, moving in the same direction as the muscle fibers.

Money-rolling is named after the gesture that indicates money or profit where a person rubs the thumb and fingers back and forth across each other. This motion is applied to areas on the body where the thumb and fingertips can grasp both sides comfortably.

C R O S S – F I B E R

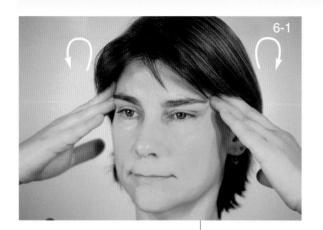

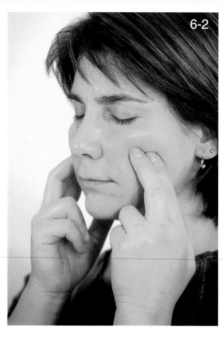

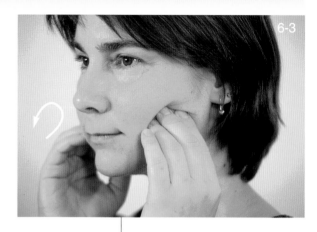

6-1, 6-2, & 6-3: You can make cross-fiber motions all over your face, using either back-and-forth movements or circles across the fibers. These three photos show several important areas where muscles tend to get tense. Different areas will need different amounts of pressure, so keep your touch light enough to make it comfortable. Rub in circles over your forehead, moving out to your temples. Your temporalis muscle fibers radiate out in a semicircle from just above the side of your cheekbone, so circles work well. Continue making circles or using a back-and-forth motion under your cheek bones, moving out to your jaw muscles toward the angle of your jaw. Experiment with different directions and pressures to see what feels best.

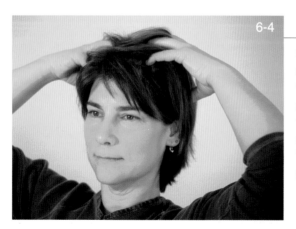

6-4: Friction for your scalp is a lot like a shampoo. (The next time you wash your hair, focus on it as not only a task to complete, but a massage that can feel wonderful!) Use your fingertips or the pads of your fingers to make short back-and-forth strokes or small circles. Then try large circles, listening for what your scalp and head like the best.

C R O S S – F I B E R

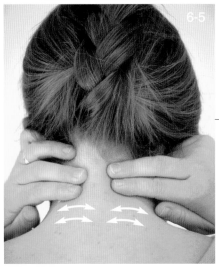

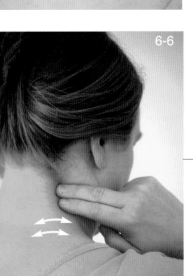

6-5 & 6-6: Walk two or three fingers up and down the back of your neck, making circles or back-and-forth movements on each side of the spine, starting at the middle, and then moving out to the edges of the vertebrae on the posterior sides of your neck. It's surprising how far out they go, so explore the back of your neck to get a feel for it. There are many important muscles bunched into a small area, so take your time when working with them. Notice what each area feels like and adjust your movements for comfort.

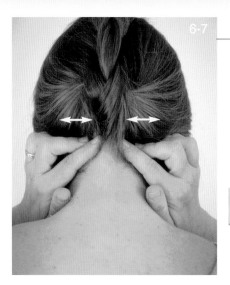

6-7: Apply pressure using short back-and-forth movements just under the base of your skull, covering the muscles, tendons and their attachments to your skull...

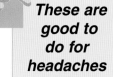

These are good to do for headaches

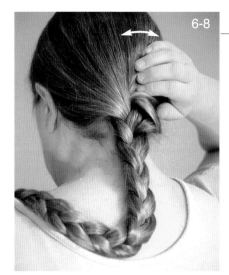

6-8: ...when you get to the attachment of the big muscle right next to your spine (the trapezius, or the "traps"), move up that muscle with side-to-side pressure; it has a long tendinous attachment that goes part way up the back of your skull. Lying down or leaning your head back as you do this will relax the muscle so it can receive the benefit more easily.

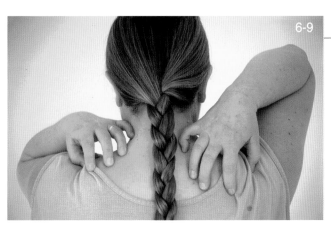

6-9: Use a strong raking motion with all four fingers, pulling your fingers across the big muscles that go from your neck across the tops of your shoulders (trapezius muscles). You can do it in an alternating manner like in this figure, or both at the same time. If you do it lying down, your muscles can relax better.

C R O S S – F I B E R

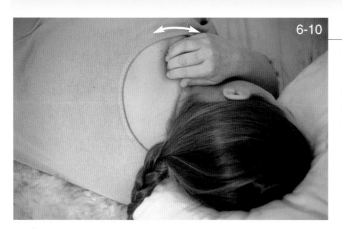

6-10: Use your fingertips to work on more specific spots in these muscles. Roll back and forth across the muscle or make small circles.

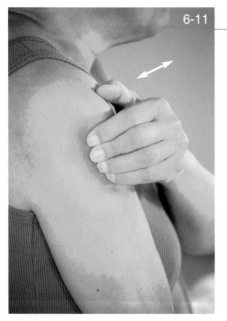

6-11: Use your fingertips to press into the muscle that goes around the top of your arm (deltoid), covering all three sections, front, side, and back. Move your fingers back and forth while pressing in toward the bone, feeling your fingers move across the muscle fibers. You can extend this stroke down your tricep muscle on the back of your upper arm.

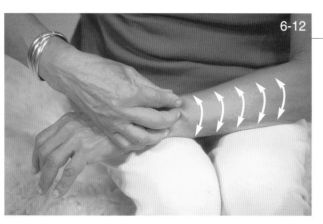

6-12: Roll your fingers back and forth over the muscles on the back of your forearm. These are the muscles that straighten your wrist and fingers, and pull your hand upward. Move from your elbow down to your wrist and glide back up.

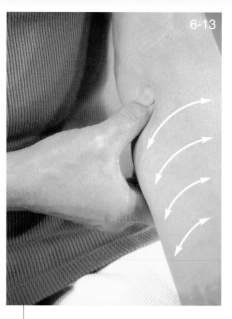

6-13: Use your thumb to do friction across the fibers of your inner forearm (the flexors that bend your fingers and wrist). An alternate way of doing this is to rest your forearm across your waist and wrap your other hand around it so your fingers can roll across the muscles in your inner forearm.

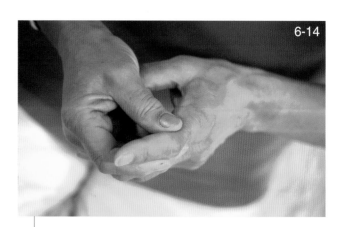

6-14: Holding each finger between the pads of your thumb and fingers, roll the tissue in a back and forth motion, both on the sides and on the top and bottom of your fingers. You can move both up and down your fingers. Experiment.

C R O S S – F I B E R

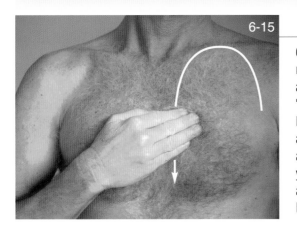

6-15: Use the pads of several fingers to make short back-and-forth motions across your upper chest, massaging your "pecs," the pectoralis major muscle. Begin where the muscle attaches on your arm (this forms the front border of your axilla or arm pit). Then move across your chest just under your collar bone and down the side of your sternum or breast bone.

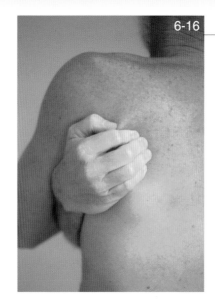

6-16: Reach around only as far and as high as is comfortable under the opposite arm onto your side and back and rub in a back-and-forth movement or in circles from the back of your shoulder (scapula) down and around your ribs. Imagine the effects moving across and down your back.

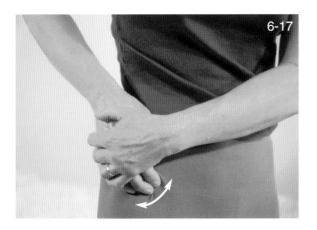

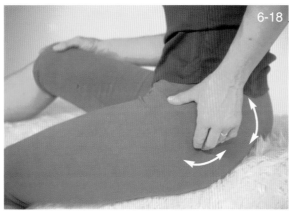

6-17 & 6-18: Sitting, standing, or lying on your side, use the pads or tips of your fingers, with your hand curved in for pressure, to roll back and forth across the muscles on the side of your hip and around the bone at the top of your leg. The fibers of these large muscles fan up and out from the greater trochanter, the bony prominence of your hip, so the angle of your cross-fiber strokes will change as you follow these muscles around.

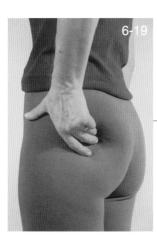

6-19: Continue exploring the large muscles in your buttock with circles, finding the bones where they attach. Begin at your sacrum or tail bone and move up and around toward the front of your hip.

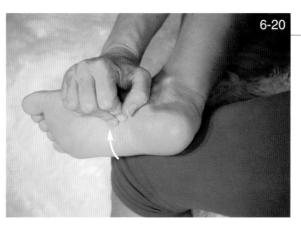

6-20: Pull your fingers across the muscles in the arch of your foot.

C I R C U L A R   T H U M B   (F I N G E R)

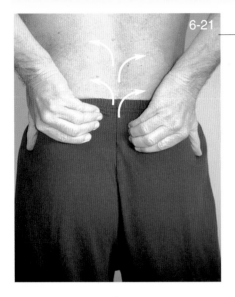

6-21: Alternating hands, make circles with your fingertips on each side of your spine, starting at your tailbone and moving only as far up your back as you can comfortably reach. This is similar to the kneading strokes for this area, but differs in that you are using the tips of your fingers in smaller, more focused circles, and the pressure is down into the muscles and tendons instead of the lifting motion with all the finger surfaces in kneading.

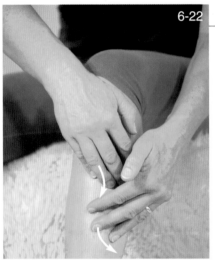

6-22: Alternating hands, use the pads of your fingers to make circles over the front of your lower leg on the lateral side of the shin bone. Move down from below your knee to your ankle, and then glide back up. You can also make small circles or do cross-fiber friction with your thumbs or fingers. Include the bony areas around the sides of your knee also, including all around your knee cap.

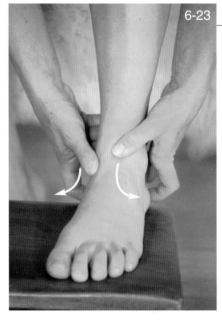

6-23: Make small circles around your ankle bones and over the top of your foot, using your thumbs or fingertips.

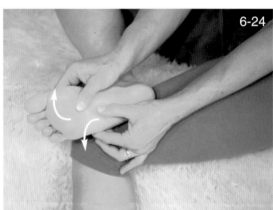

6-24: Use your thumbs to make circles all over the sole of your foot. Use the amount of pressure your feet like the best. Foot reflexology is based on the idea that certain spots on the soles of your feet (and palms of your hands, and your ears) are connected to different areas and organs in your body. Take your time to cover every bit of your foot, including your toes and the sides of your heel, knowing it will also relax and stimulate the rest of your body, too.

D E E P - F O C U S E D   G L I D E

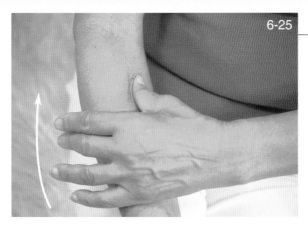

6-25: Use the tips of your fingers or thumb to make several deep-focused glide strokes up the muscles on your inner forearm. You can learn to feel the separate long tendons with relatively narrow muscles that run from the wrist to the inner side of your elbow.

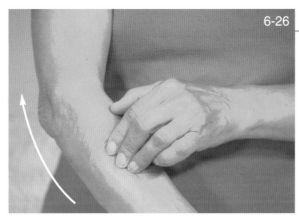

6-26: Use your fingertips to glide up the long tendons and muscles on the outside of your forearm, up to the common attachment on the bone at your elbow several times to cover all the muscles.

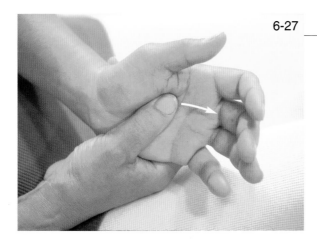

6-27: Supporting the back of your hand with your fingers, glide your thumb in strips from the heel of your palm to the base of your fingers. You can glide on top of the tendon to each finger and also between the tendons. Do this at the amount of pressure your hand likes the best. Reflexology is based on the principle that each part of the hand (and foot and ear) relates to a part of the body, and calms and helps to heal that area. So the rest of your body may feel more relaxed from this, also.

D E E P - F O C U S E D   G L I D E

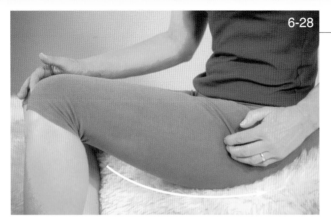

6-28: Use your fingertips with your fingers curved to glide up the wide band on the outside of your thigh between your knee and the greater trochanter (the bony prominence you feel at the top of your leg). This band is wide and fibrous, and does well with attention to its front and back edges, also. You can press into it with quite a bit of pressure unless it has tender spots. Stop at these and give some gentle massage.

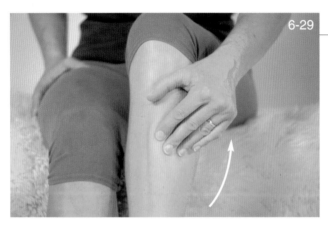

6-29: Glide your fingertips up the front of your lower leg, on the lateral side of the shin bone, the tibia. Do this several times. You can also glide up the outside of your lower leg. This will treat muscles that help stabilize your ankle. These may be tender if you have twisted or sprained your ankle in the past.

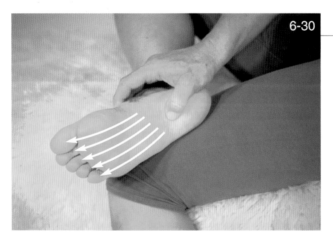

6-30: Use your thumb to glide up the sole of your foot, using the amount of pressure your foot likes best. Repeat this in narrow strips to cover the whole surface.

M O N E Y   R O L L I N G

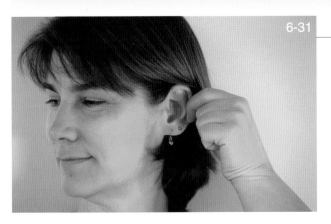

6-31: Grasp the edges of your ears between your fingertips and tip of your thumb. Move your fingers and thumb back and forth in opposite directions a couple of times, and then move on around to cover your whole ear this way. This is invigorating and relaxing. In reflexology, different parts of the ear are said to correspond to different parts of the body, so this may be very relaxing and comforting.

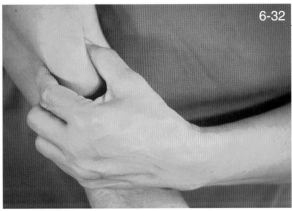

6-32: Grasp your bicep muscle on your upper arm with your fingers and thumb, and move them back and forth in opposite directions, as you move down the muscle. Glide back up.

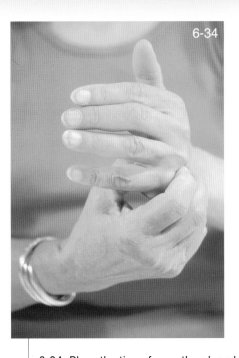

6-34: Place the tips of your thumb and fingers on opposite sides of your hand between each of the hand bones (metacarpals) and move back and forth in opposite directions. Explore the area from mid-palm (the lowest you can get into these spaces) to the webs between your fingers.

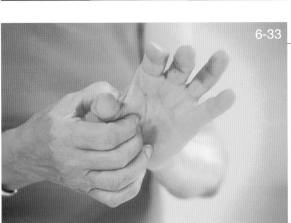

6-33: Using the tips of your thumb and first two or three fingers, grasp the area between your other thumb and first metacarpal (the bone in the hand below your first finger) and rock them back and forth over this fleshy muscle. Explore the whole space, noticing how the muscles are shaped and how much pressure they enjoy.

Remember to note your preferences for strokes in your journal.

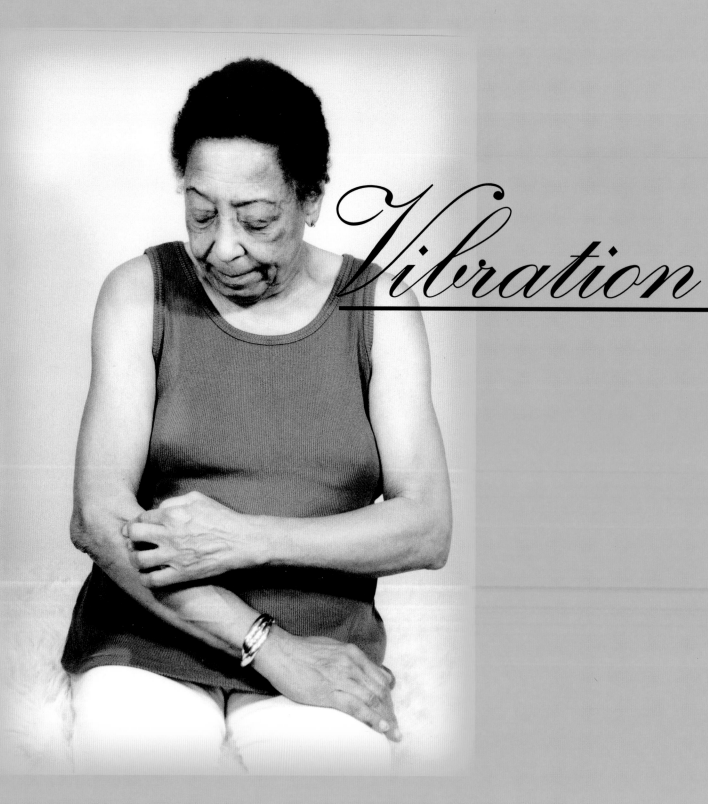

Vibration

Chapter 7 – Vibration

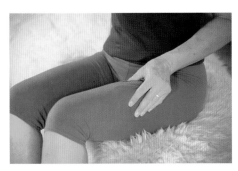

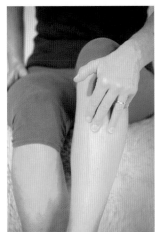

VIBRATION and JOSTLING strokes are relaxing and calming. They soften and loosen superficial tissues and muscles and activate the part of the autonomic nervous system that brings us into an overall state of rest and calm. Vibration and jostling strokes also relax the peripheral nerves that go to the arms, legs, and surface of the body. They are good strokes to use after a more vigorous or specifically focused massage, as they bring the tissues back to rest.

Jostling shakes a muscle back and forth, using your fingertips or the pads of your fingers. It works best for long muscles, since the muscle body is freer to move sideways than in shorter muscles. You will use this stroke primarily for muscles in your arms and legs. Place your fingertips on the middle of a muscle and rapidly shake them back and forth with a gentle firmness. Or you can shake the muscle between your fingertips and thumb.

Vibration uses a continuous shaking or trembling of your hands or fingers to create a rapid shaking of superficial or deep tissues anywhere on the body. For self-massage, use an approach that "makes waves" down the muscle you are working on. It feels wonderfully relaxing and stimulating at the same time. Use your fingers in a side-to-side vibration or shaking movement. Place all your fingertips on the skin at one end of the area you are working on; then shake them back and forth rapidly while moving your hand along the muscle or limb. If this stroke left tracks on the skin it would look like a row of waves.

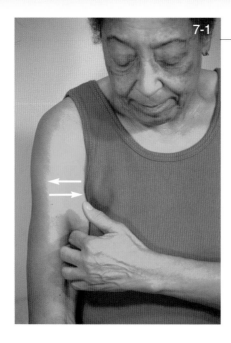

7-1: Place your fingertips right on top of your bicep muscle in your upper arm and jostle it back and forth by shaking your fingers across the muscle rapidly.

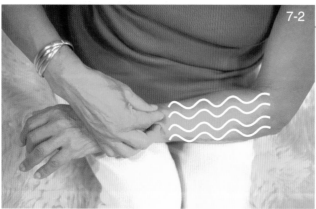

7-2: Rest your arm across your lap, palm down. Vibrate the muscles on the back of your forearm by lightly placing your fingertips just below your elbow and shaking them back and forth as you pull your fingers down your arm. If you left tracks on your arm, they'd look like several sets of parallel waves. Turn the palm of your receiving arm up, and "make waves" for the inside of your forearm too.

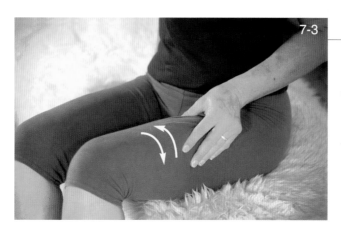

7-3: Lightly grasp your thigh muscles between your fingers and thumb. Shake the muscle back and forth rapidly.

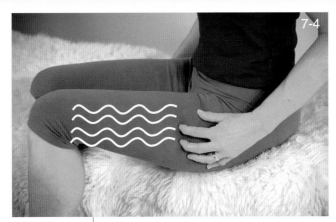

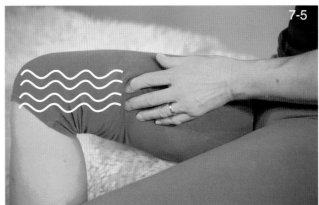

7-4 & 7-5: Use the pads of your fingers to make vibration waves over each side of your thigh, moving from knee to hip. Do them several times if you like them. Experiment with the style of vibration your legs enjoy the most.

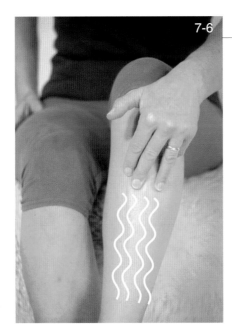

7-6 Make waves up your lower leg from ankle to knee. Experiment with doing this on all sides of your lower leg, noticing how your muscles feel in response.

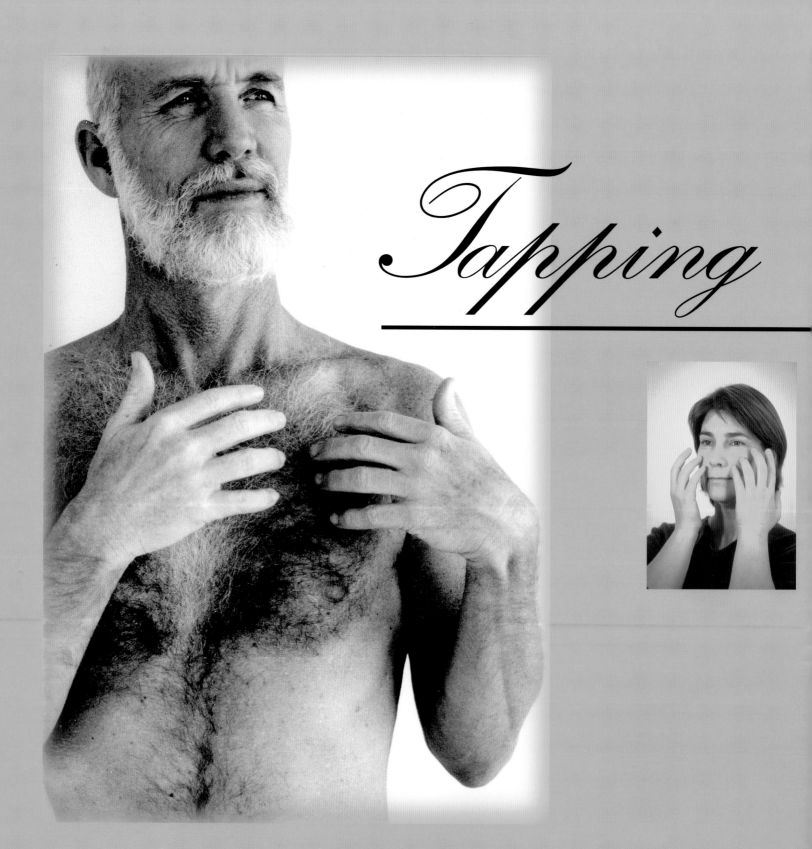

Tapping

Chapter 8 - *Tapping*

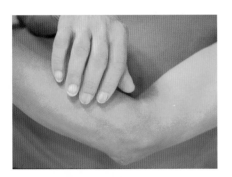

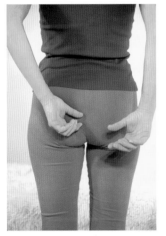

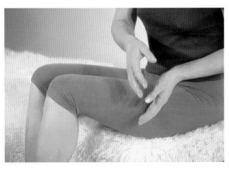

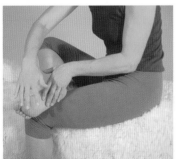

*T*APPING or tapotement is a percussive movement, typically using both hands to alternately strike the tissue. The hands must remain soft and relaxed, giving a light and smooth movement that comes from the wrist. Use this only over well-protected areas that don't have abnormally contracted muscles, for example, not on the low back or abdomen. You can adapt this to be used with one hand for your own self-massage. One woman in my self-massage group is very creative with this, drumming her fingers over her arm or leg with a gentle touch; it's very soothing to watch.

The benefits of tapping include stimulating your body systems and relieving congested areas. It stretches the muscles at the brief time they are being tapped, and then lets them relax between the taps. This rapid alternation of stretching and shortening seems to help the muscles to settle into a softer, more relaxed state; at the same time it invigorates them. It improves circulation; the skin will often get pink from the increased blood flow.

Drumming, a very gentle tapping of the fingers, can be used over the sinus areas in the cheeks and forehead to help relieve congestion. A gentle drumming over any area of your body is very relaxing. Over larger, protected areas you can use more force.

Tapping can be done with the fingertips and is usually used in a smaller area. You can use both hands or one hand for this rapid stroke. When using both hands you can alternate them or strike the skin simultaneously. For one hand or simultaneous use of both hands, watch the tissue to see when it bounces back from the tapping; time your tapping to occur just as the tissue gets back to its original shape.

Don't do this over your low back because it is not a protected area (there's no bony shell protecting the organs). The kidneys are in this area and you can damage them.

Beating is done by shaping your hand into a loose fist and beating with the side of your hand with a loose wrist. This is good for a large area such as your buttocks. When doing it for yourself, you'll beat with the thumb side of your hand for your buttocks, and the fifth finger side for your legs.

Hacking is a stroke with which you may be familiar. One person does a rapid tapping of another's shoulders and back with the fifth-finger side of the hands. It can look like it's a hard strike of the tissue, but since the hand and wrist are relaxed, it does not hurt or give too much of a challenge to the tissue. When doing this stroke, you will know you are doing it right if you feel your fingers slapping together in a loose way each time you strike the tissue.

Slapping can feel great, especially over the feet and legs. It is stimulating and relaxing at the same time. Again, it is done with a soft hand and wrist, letting your fingers slap your skin.

D R U M M I N G / T A P P I N G

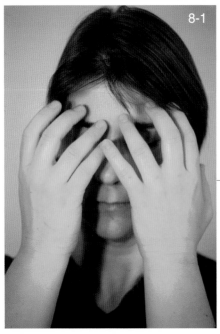

8-1

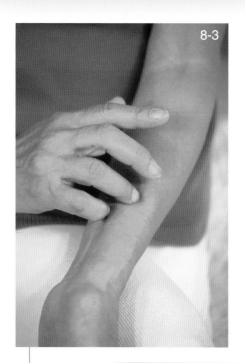

8-3

8-1 & 8-2: Using a very gentle touch, drum your fingers over your bony sinus areas on your forehead and cheeks. Simply let your relaxed fingers rapidly fall against your skin one at a time, from 5th to 1st finger and bounce right off. If you have any congestion, these areas can be very tender, so do this lightly, with subtlety. It can help sinuses drain and relieve pressure if you don't do it too hard. Also experiment with drumming over the muscles in your cheeks and jaw. You may also find that your temples and scalp like this stroke.

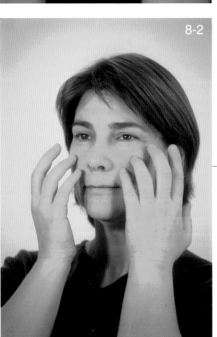

8-2

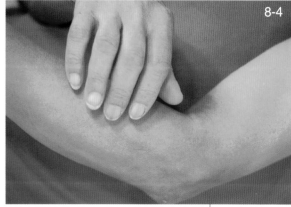

8-4

8-3 & 8-4: You can tap all over your arm, using either a drumming motion as shown above in photo 8-3, or by tapping all four fingers at once as in photo 8-4. Keep your hand and fingers soft and relaxed, and let your fingertips or flat fingers fall onto the surface of your arm, lifting them immediately as if you are bouncing off the surface like a springy ball. Experiment with the pacing and with the vigor you use in tapping. Also try this for your hands, too.

Chapter 8 – Tapping

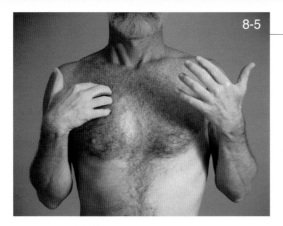

8-5: Use the fingertips of both hands to tap alternately, moving across your chest, avoiding any breast tissue. Keeping your hand and fingers soft and relaxed, bounce your fingertips easily against your chest. Experiment with your pacing and pressure. You can keep your hands next to each other or tap on both sides of your chest at the same time. Find what works best for you.

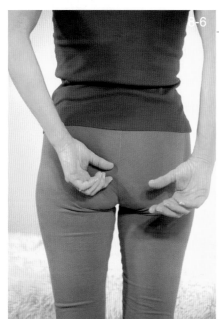

8-6: Form a loose fist and beat across your buttocks, with hands and wrists loose and flexible. Bounce back off instantly and cover your whole buttock and hip area. Notice it is the thumb side of your hand that contacts the skin.

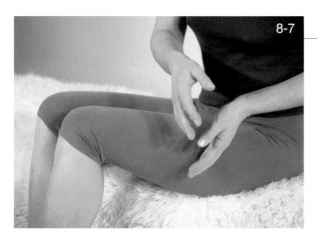

8-7: Again keeping your hands and fingers loose, use a rapid hacking motion for your thighs, alternately striking the muscles with the fifth-finger side of each hand. Keep your hands, fingers, and wrists loose, so that you can hear and feel your fingers slapping against each other each time your hand contacts your leg.

T A P P I N G & S L A P P I N G

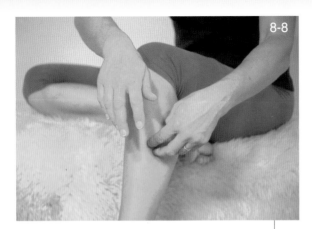

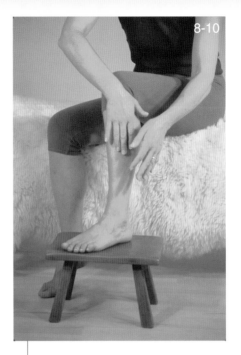

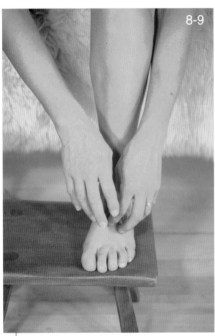

8-8 & 8-9: Continue tapping over your lower leg and foot, alternately tapping the fingertips of each hand against the muscles and tendons around the leg, ankle, and foot. Experiment with speed and pressure, expecting that different spots will like different things best.

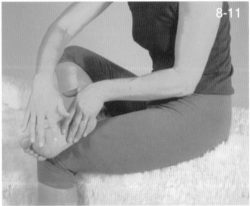

8-10 & 8-11: Slapping with relaxed hands is another style of tapping; some people enjoy this a lot, and others don't. Experiment with this for your lower leg and foot. Keeping your hands soft, begin with a gentle, rapid slapping motion as you move across your leg and foot. This can be invigorating and pleasant. If it's not, go back to massage strokes you like. If it feels good, experiment with it for other areas of your body. Note preferences in your journal.

Chapter 9
Whole Body Relaxation Massage

his chapter leads you through a whole body massage for overall relaxation. The intention of this massage is to relax your whole body when you feel stressed or weary. This self-massage process is presented through photographs and brief instructions. For more detailed information refer back to Chapters 4 through 8. The KindTouch CD includes a half-hour self-massage to help you learn the sequence and strokes. Below is a quick reference summarizing the five strokes.

SUMMARY OF THE FIVE STROKES

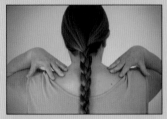

GLIDING
In gliding, make long smooth strokes in the direction of the muscle fibers, molding your hands or fingers to the body contours. In general, heavier pressure goes toward the heart, lighter pressure can go either direction.

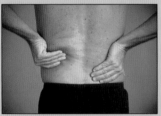

KNEADING OR SQUEEZING
In kneading, conform your hands or fingers to the tissue and lift, squeeze, and knead it away from the underlying structure. You can use one or two hands, using the flats of your fingers, lifting them toward the heel of your hand or your flat thumb in a firm circular motion. Start at the area closest to the heart and gradually move down the limb or area you're working on. Always follow with a firm, gliding stroke toward your heart.

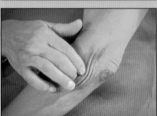

FRICTION
In friction strokes, compress the tissue with your fingers, thumbs, or hands, moving the more surface layers over the underlying structures. It's a more focused stroke than the others and generally moves across the direction of the muscle fibers. Always follow friction with gliding.

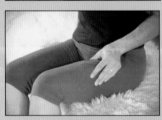

VIBRATION
Vibration strokes shake or vibrate the tissue. One way to do vibration is to grasp the muscle and shake it back and forth. Another is to "make waves" down a muscle by placing the fingertips over one end of the muscle and shaking them back and forth while moving them along the length of the muscle.

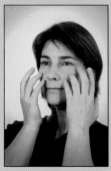

TAPPING
Tapping is done only over areas with bones under them, that is, not the low back or abdomen. Tapping is a percussive movement using very relaxed hands or fingers. On the face, it is done very lightly, using only the fingers. Otherwise, the movement is from the wrist and is light and smooth.

Each time you give yourself a massage, refer to your journal notes, remember the approach that each part of your body likes, and listen for cues about different ways each area would like to be touched. The photographs are merely reminders of sequences; use your own body wisdom to choose strokes and how to apply them. Add reminders in your journal as you make discoveries.

Massage therapists learn how important it is to be conscious of how we begin a massage and how we move from stroke to stroke. I always begin with gentle gliding strokes; it not only spreads the oil but begins the connection between the one who is giving the massage and the one who is receiving it. This is a vital step and sets the direction, quality, and depth of communication for the bodywork.

In self-massage this is an essential step also, as it brings your focus inward, releasing the often racing preoccupations of your mind. This true connection can be even more complex in self-massage, since you are both giving and receiving the touch. It is easy to lose your open-hearted connection with yourself if you merely go straight to the sore spot and try to "rub it out." When you set the stage in a conscious and respectful manner, the effects of your self-massage will be much deeper.

Chapter 9 – Whole Body Relaxation Massage

The first touch in a massage gets your muscles and tissues used to your touch. Attention to a whole area with gliding can cut down on the amount of focused work needed by starting to soften the whole area. When an area is injured, the muscles surrounding it become tight and guarded; this is a protective mechanism that "splints" the injured area to avoid sudden movements and pain. Unfortunately, this causes the surrounding muscles to be sore and restricted, also. Beginning massage by gently working over the whole area calms all the muscles, and provides good support to the injured area by letting it rest in a gentle container of relaxed muscles. The sequence of strokes tends to move from gentle and broad movements to deeper and more specific work.

A typical Swedish massage sequence is as follows:

1. **Gentle gliding with oil**
2. **Deeper gliding**
3. **Kneading**
4. **Gliding**
5. **Friction**
6. **Gliding**
7. **Vibration or tapping**
8. **Gliding**
9. **Nerve strokes (very light gliding)**

Notice how many times gliding is used. It is a great transition stroke, helping the tissues soak in the direct muscular effects of each of the other strokes; and it also builds on the benefits from the other strokes that improve circulation and lymphatic flow to remove waste products and bring in healthy nutrients.

Accept your body. If you have a certain idea about how the body should be, you will be in misery...If you start loving it, you will find it is changing, because if a person loves his body he starts taking care, and care implies everything.

Osho

WHOLE BODY RELAXATION MASSAGE

Exercise 9

Introduction

You will be giving yourself a whole body relaxation massage in this exercise. So far you have learned how to do each stroke. Now you will learn how to put them together for a complete massage. You can use one of two approaches; each will familiarize you with the way strokes are combined. You can follow the one-half hour Guided Self-Massage on the *KindTouch CD*, or follow the photographic sequences in the book. The photographs give a good visual overview of a complete massage. The book reviews all the strokes, while the CD guides you through the strokes most easily combined for a complete massage in one-half hour.

Preparation

Begin by gathering massage oil or wearing comfortable, non-binding, unbulky clothes; remove jewelry; and fasten long hair off of your neck. Set up a warm, comfortable area where you won't be interrupted. If you are using oil, protect your chair or bed with a sheet or towel, and place the oil bottle on a saucer in case of drips. Have a stool to rest your feet on for massaging your legs, or sit on your bed, couch, or floor.

If you use the guided massage on the CD, have the remote control for the CD player handy so that if you find tender areas or want to spend more time working on any part of your body, you can pause the CD at that point. Or you can return to that area after the massage. Use the first time through to get a sense of it. It will become familiar with practice.

If you follow the photographs in the book, you will find all the strokes demonstrated. You can choose the ones you like the best for each part of your body, spending as much time as you like in each area. You may want to play relaxing music you enjoy.

DIRECTIONS

1. Choose to follow the one-half hour guided massage on the *KindTouch CD* or to follow the photographic sequence in the book.
2. If you choose the CD, you may want to scan the photographic sequences in this chapter first to acquaint yourself with the sequence of strokes for the head-to-toe massage.
3. If you follow the book, begin by listening to the *Self-Blessing* or by taking eight deep breaths to calm and center your body, mind, heart, and soul.
4. Remember that all strokes are included and, following the photographs and directions, choose the strokes you like best for each part of your body.

5. When you start, begin with smooth gliding whether you are using oil or not, and use the time to slow down and come present. This will allow you to bring your heart, mind and soul into your hands so they can give the gift of a listening and healing touch to your body. Your attention is called to your body and its sensations, and also to your hands as communication tools between your body and your heart, mind, and soul.
6. Complete the self-massage with open-heartedness in both giving and receiving.
7. Record your experience in your journal.

Journal

- How do you feel now, compared to before your massage?
- What did you enjoy most about the massage you gave yourself? What's the best thing about your touch?
- What was easy, and what was a challenge?
- Were you able to experience both giving and receiving? Where and when was it easiest, and most difficult?
- What areas wanted more time? How will you adapt this massage for yourself in the future?

This Week and Beyond

- Give yourself another self-massage in the next week, and notice how your comfort with the sequences deepens.
- As you become familiar with doing this massage, place more of your attention on the inside of your body and muscles, noticing how they receive the touch.
- Spend more time massaging the areas that want more touch.
- Find the times you can add self-massage informally. For example, while lying awake in the night, when relaxing in the evening, during brief breaks from typing at the computer or from any kind of work you are doing, while you are thinking about what you will do next, and so on. Make your own list.

...You only have to let the soft animal of your body love what it loves...

Mary Oliver

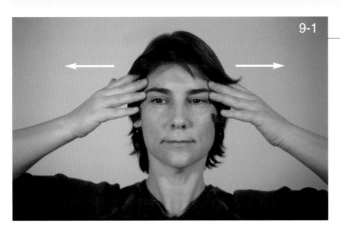

9-1: Glide across your forehead several times, ending with circles over your temples.

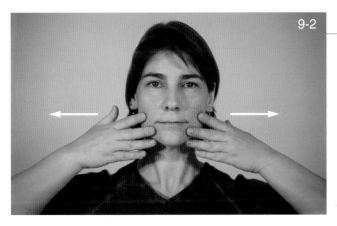

9-2: Glide across your cheeks and chin several times, ending with circles over your jaw muscles.

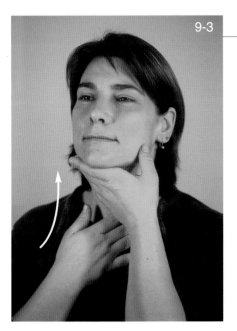

9-3: Glide up your throat several times, alternating hands.

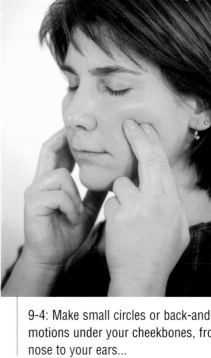

9-4: Make small circles or back-and-forth motions under your cheekbones, from your nose to your ears...

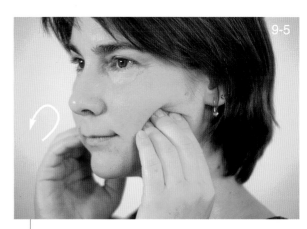

9-5: ...and then across your cheeks, above your jaw line, and out to the corner of your jaw. Continue until you feel your jaw muscles soften.

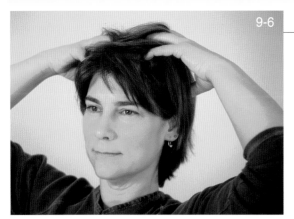

9-6: Shampoo your scalp with your fingertips, making circles or back-and-forth motions.

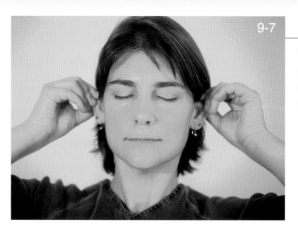

9-7: Money-roll your ears, squeezing each spot between your thumb and finger(s).

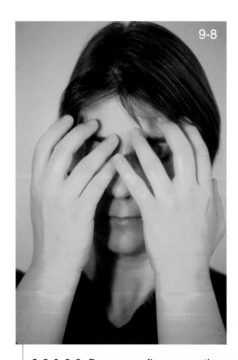

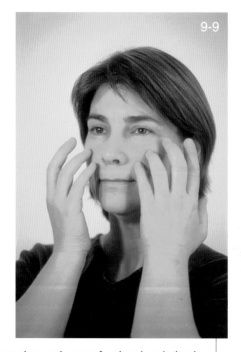

9-8 & 9-9: Drum your fingers gently over your sinuses in your forehead and cheeks.

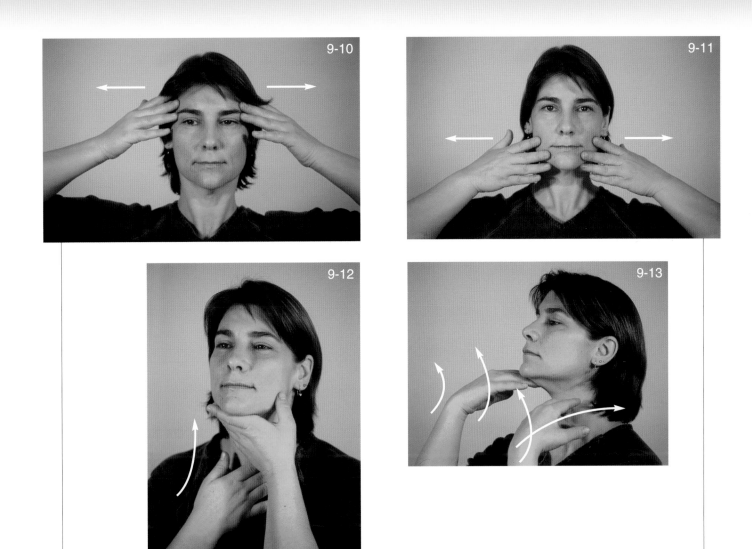

9-10, 9-11, 9-12, & 9-13: Finish by gliding over your whole face again, and doing nerve strokes over your face and neck.

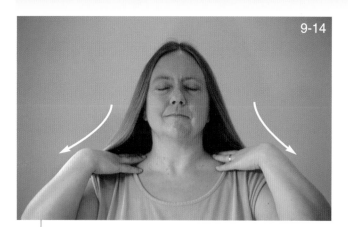

9-14: Glide down your neck and across your shoulders several times...

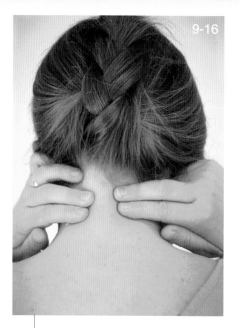

9-16: Walk your fingers down your neck, making friction circles or back-and-forth motions, starting toward the center of your neck....

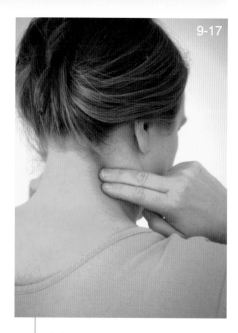

9-17: ...and moving out toward the sides of your neck.

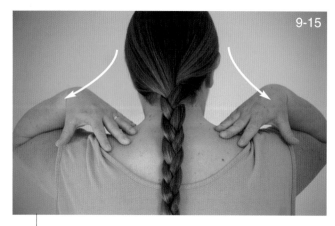

9-15: ...making sure to cover the back of your neck and shoulders also.

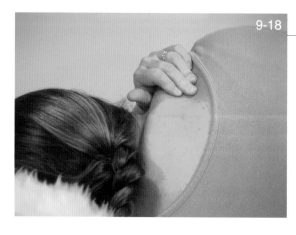

9-18: Keep moving down to your upper shoulders, kneading them either between your fingers and the heel of your hand...

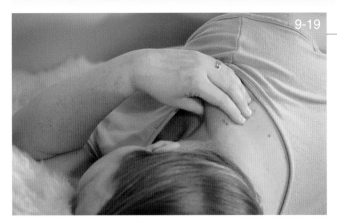

9-19: ...or between your fingers and thumb.

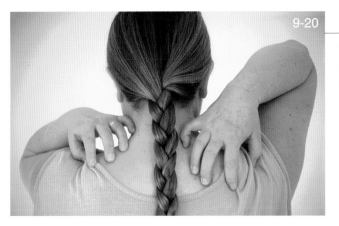

9-20: Rake your fingers over your upper shoulders, and then...

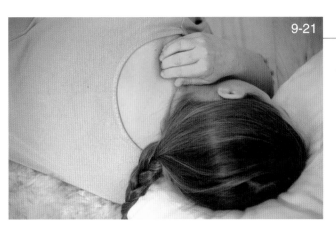

9-21: ...use the tips of your fingers to focus on tight spots with friction circles or back-and-forth movements.

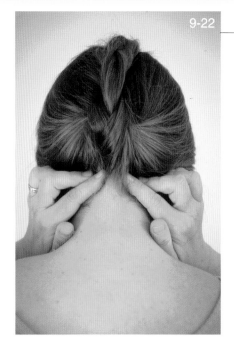

9-22: Do cross-fiber friction all across the base of your skull...

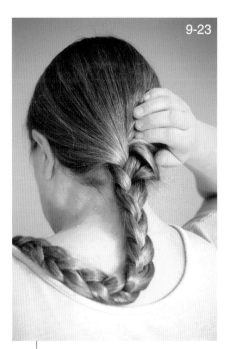

9-23: ...then continue friction up onto the tendons over the lower part of your skull.

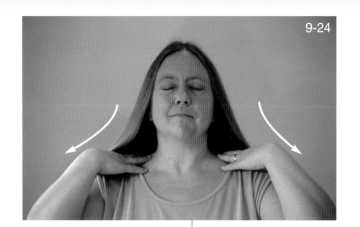

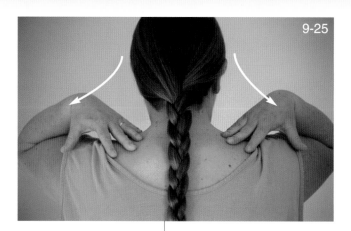

9-24 & 9-25: Finish by gliding over your neck and shoulders...

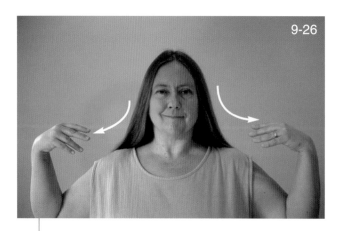

9-26: ...and end with nerve strokes.

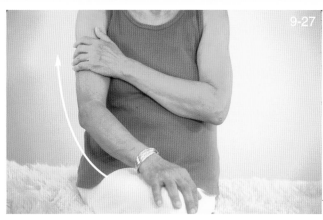

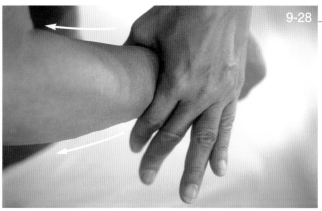

9-27 & 9-28: Glide up each side of your arm several times.

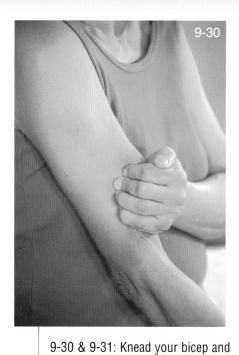

9-30 & 9-31: Knead your bicep and tricep muscles on the front and back of your upper arm, working down to your elbow, and gliding back up.

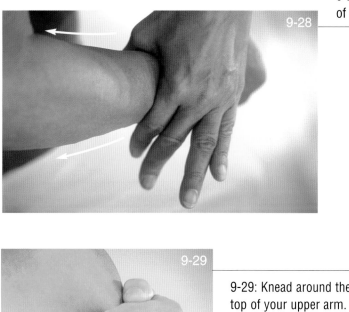

9-29: Knead around the top of your upper arm.

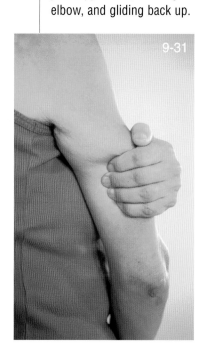

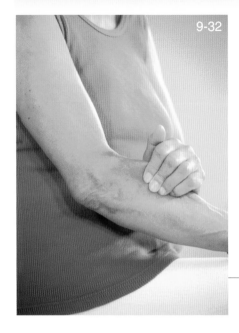

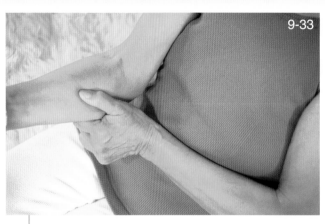

9-32 & 9-33: Knead all sides of your forearm, working from elbow to wrist and gliding back up.

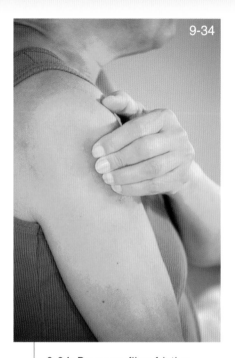

9-34: Do cross-fiber friction around the top of your upper arm, then move down the back of your arm and glide back up.

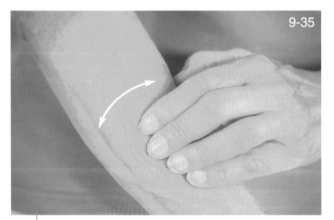

9-35 & 9-36: Roll back and forth across the muscles in your forearm, front and back, gliding back up your whole arm.

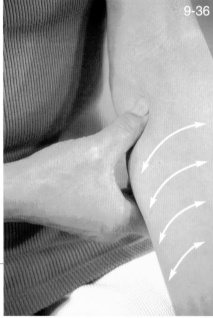

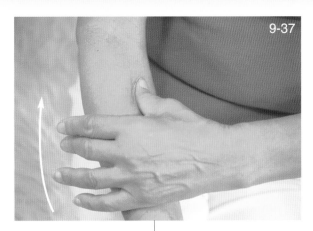 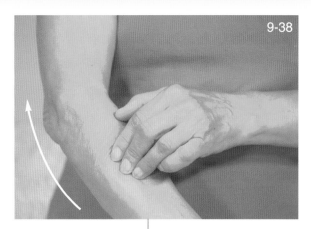

9-37 & 9-38: Do focused gliding several times up the long tendons and muscles on the inside and outside of your forearm, and then knead and glide up to settle the muscles.

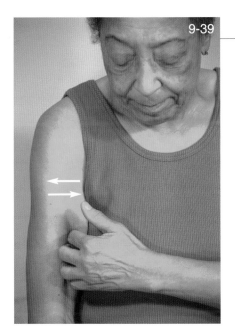

9-39: Jostle the muscles in your upper arm.

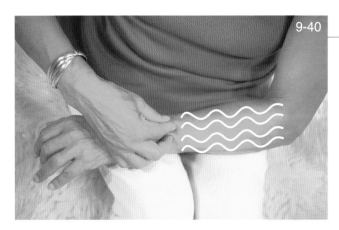

9-40: Make vibration waves down your forearm and glide back up your whole arm.

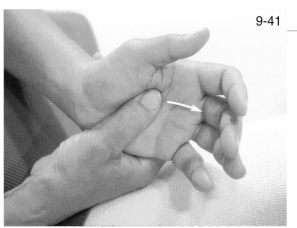

9-41: Glide down the palm of your hand along the tendons to each finger and also between them.

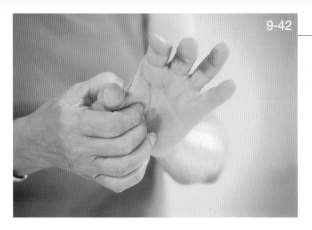

9-42: Money-roll the tissue between your thumb and hand.

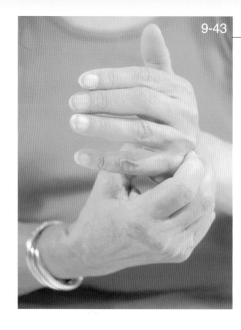

9-43: Money-roll the tissue between the bones going to each finger.

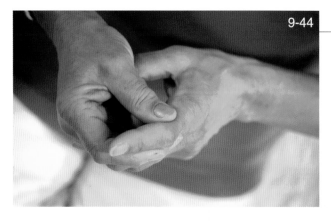

9-44: Roll each finger between your thumb and fingers, covering all sides with cross-fiber friction.

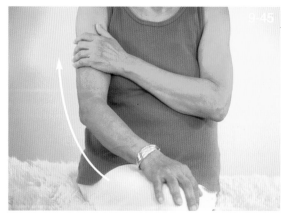

9-45: Finish by gliding up all surfaces of your arm...

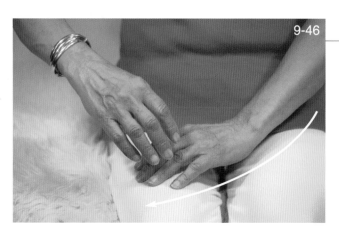

9-46: ...and end with nerve strokes.

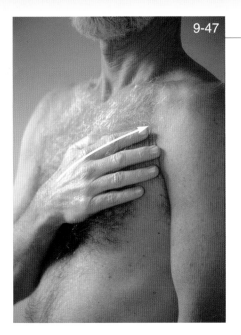

9-47: Glide out over your chest and down over your side.

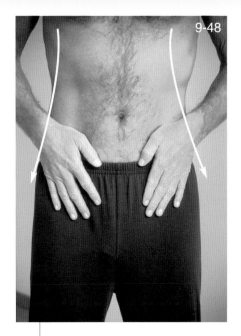

9-48: Glide down over your abdomen to your hips.

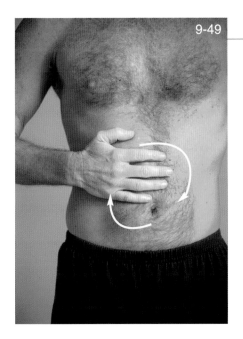

9-49: Glide in a circle around your abdomen, making sure you move up the right side, across below the ribs, and down the left side so you go with your bowel, not against it.

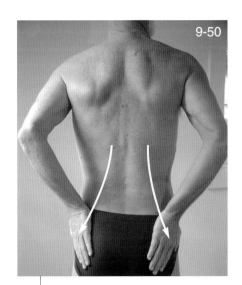

9-50: Glide down your back, going only as far as you can comfortably reach.

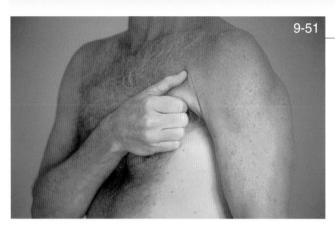

9-51: Knead your chest, gliding back up...

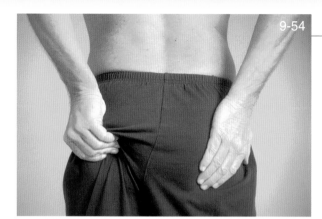

9-54: ...and continue down to knead your hips and buttocks. Then glide over these muscles.

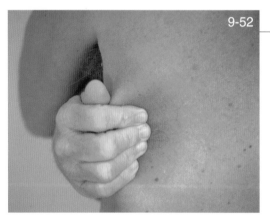

9-52: ...then move around and knead the muscles on your side as far around onto your back as you can comfortably reach.

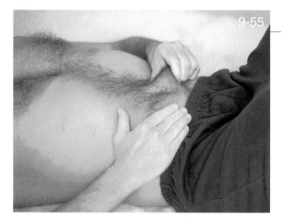

9-55: Lying down, you can knead your abdominal muscles...

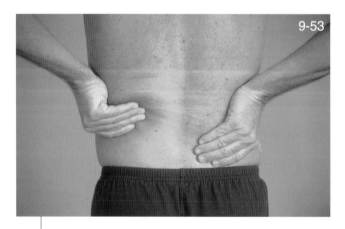

9-53: Knead your lower back...

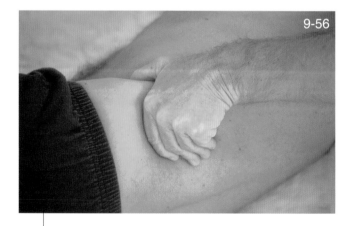

9-56: ...then roll to your side and knead the muscles at the side of your waist.

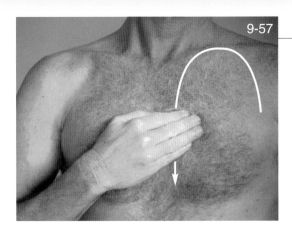

9-57: Using your fingertips, do cross-fiber friction from the inside of your upper arm, around under your collar bone, and down the side of your breast bone.

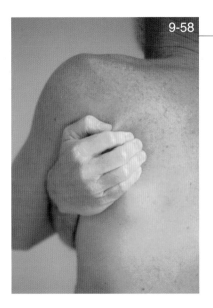

9-58: Reach around and do cross-fiber friction over the muscles on your back.

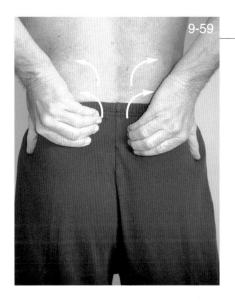

9-59: Do circular friction from your tailbone as far up your back as is comfortable.

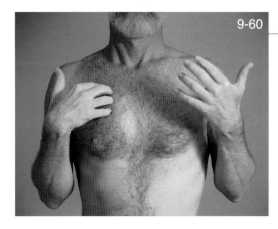

9-60: Tap alternate hands over your chest.

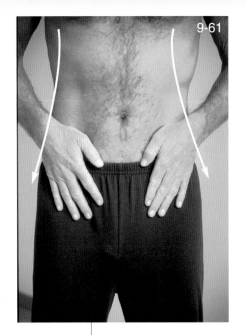
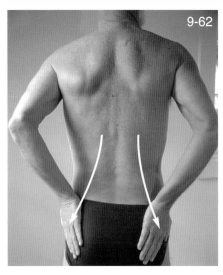
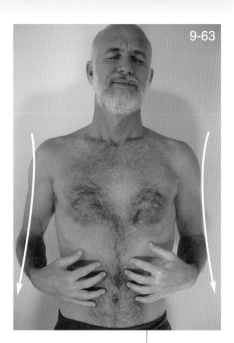

9-61, 9-62, & 9-63: Finish by gliding over the front and back of your torso, and doing nerve strokes.

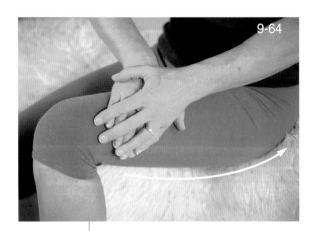
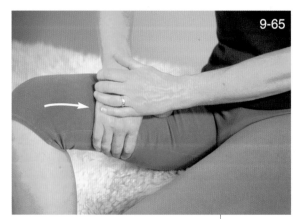

9-64 & 9-65: Glide up all sides of your thigh, using two hands for firmer pressure.

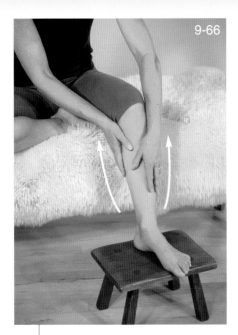

9-66: Glide up both sides of your lower leg.

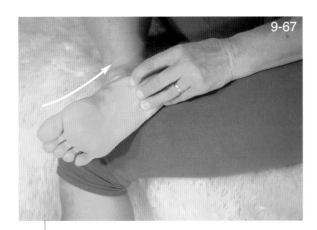

9-67: Glide up the sole of your foot.

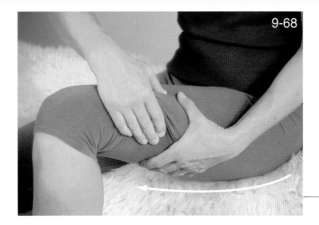

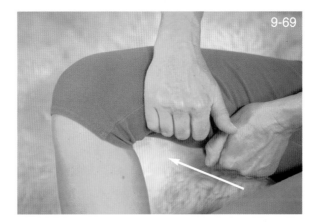

9-68, 9-69, & 9-70: Knead all sides of your thigh from hip to knee, and glide back up.

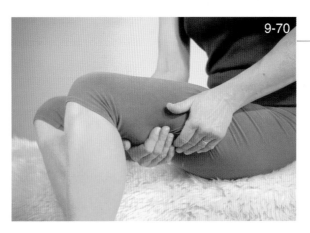

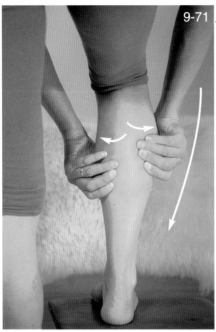

9-71: Knead the back of your calf with one or two hands and glide back up.

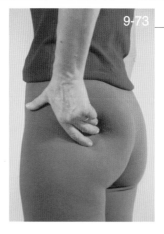

9-73: Explore the large muscles in your buttock with back-and-forth motions or circles.

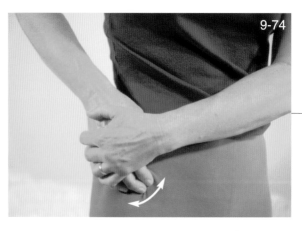

9-74: Do cross-fiber friction over the side of your hip between your waist and lateral hip bone.

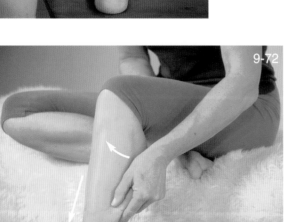

9-72: Knead the side of your calf with one hand.

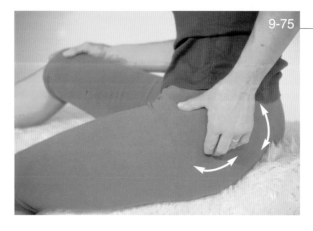

9-75: Work your way around the bony prominence at the side of your hip with friction circles or back-and-forth motions.

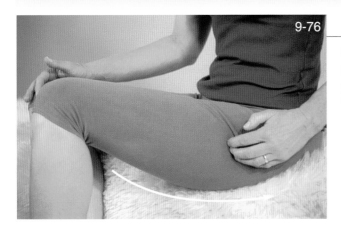

9-76: Do a deep focused glide up the outside of your thigh from knee to hip.

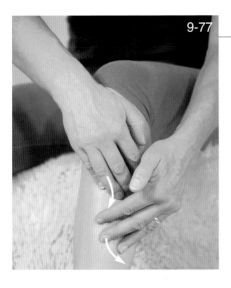

9-77: Make friction circles as you move down your lower leg.

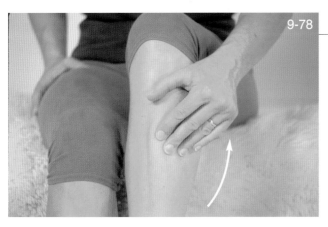

9-78: Do a deep-focused glide up the muscle just to the side of the bone in the front of your lower leg.

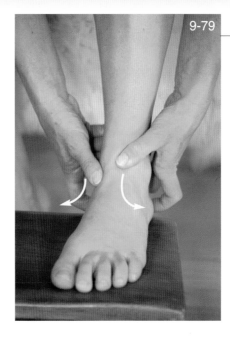

9-79: Do circular thumb friction around your ankle...

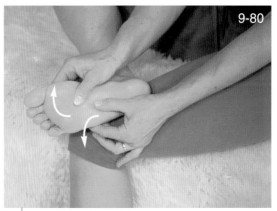

9-80: ...and over the whole sole of your foot.

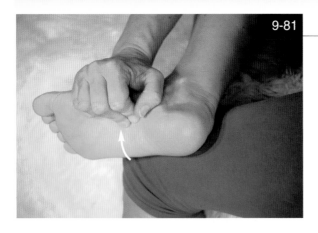

9-81: Do cross-fiber friction across the arch of your foot.

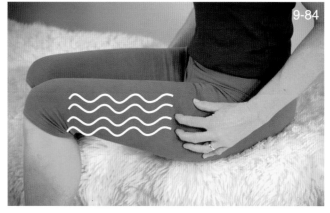

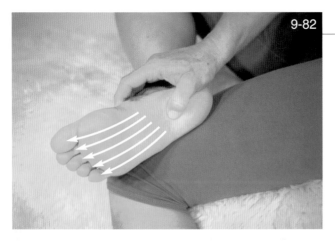

9-82: Run your thumb from your heel to your toes in strips to cover the whole surface.

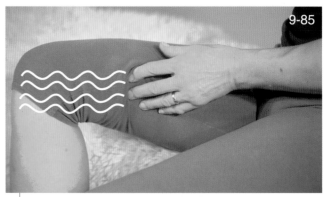

9-84 & 9-85: Vibrate both sides of your thigh by making waves with your fingers.

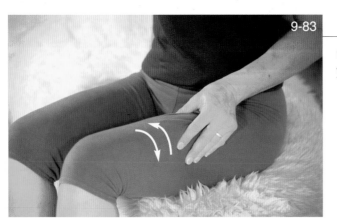

9-83: Jostle the front of your thigh.

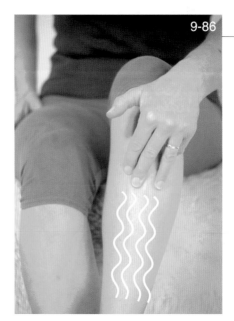

9-86: Vibrate your leg by making waves with your fingers as you pull your hand from your ankle to your knee.

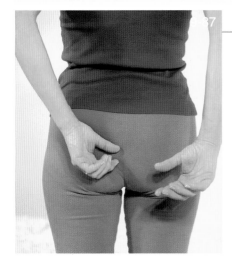

9-87: Beat your hips and buttocks with a loose fist.

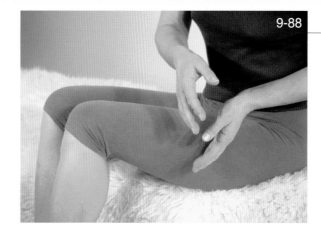

9-88: Hack your thighs with loose hands.

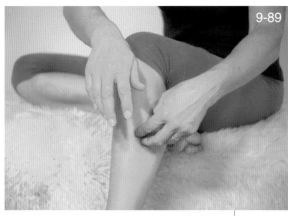

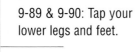

9-89 & 9-90: Tap your lower legs and feet.

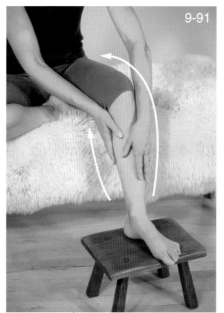

9-91 & 9-92: Finish by gliding over your whole leg and then doing nerve strokes.

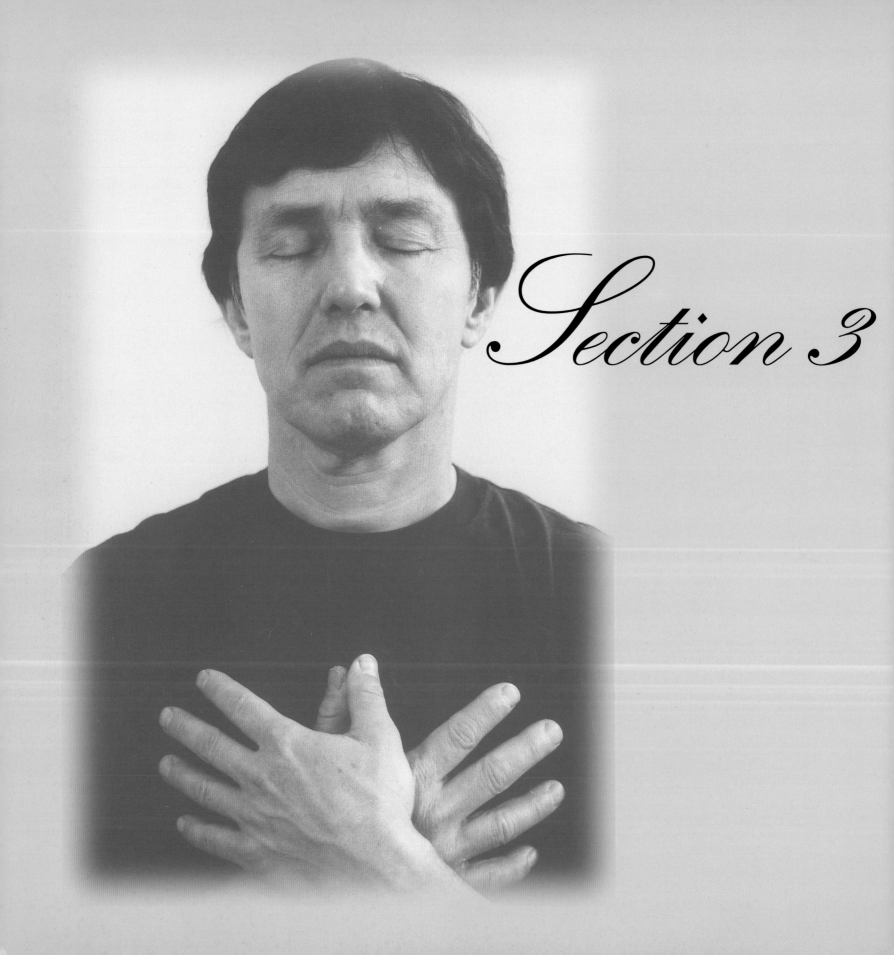

Section 3

Moving Into Healing

he road toward healing is often not apparent when we are in a crisis or feeling ill. Just when we need it the most, the healing path may seem the most elusive. Fortunately, our bodies can give us the direction to move in. KindTouch gives us something we can do when we don't know what to do.

Self-massage gives us a means of deepening our ability to hear subtle messages from our bodies and to soften into a supportive, loving response. Focusing our attention through our hands helps us to be present for ourselves. This is a powerful gift. Then we deepen our experience of wholeness—body, mind, heart, and soul.

Self-massage includes every part of a person. The mind, heart, and soul are the givers and the body is the receiver. As our bodies relax into KindTouch, our hearts also soften with the joy and contentment that come when we receive loving care. The giving and receiving roles then begin to blur, and the gifts the body receives are returned to the rest of the whole person, calming and healing each level of our beings.

This experience of wholeness makes it possible to love and accept all of ourselves, the difficult along with the pleasant. As we come to know and accept ourselves more fully, we are able to find a better balance in our lives that supports our unique selves.

We support healing in ourselves through our choices. Choosing to move toward healing and wholeness allows us to reclaim parts of ourselves we've rejected or ignored, and helps us to remain unbroken in the face of new illness, injury, or loss. In order to move toward wholeness, we must stop and face the wound and learn how to be open and care for it and ourselves kindly. KindTouch gives us a gentle path to follow in this healing challenge.

Always look at what happens when you do something: if you become peaceful, if you become restful, at home, relaxed, it is right. This is the criterion, nothing else is the criterion.

Osho

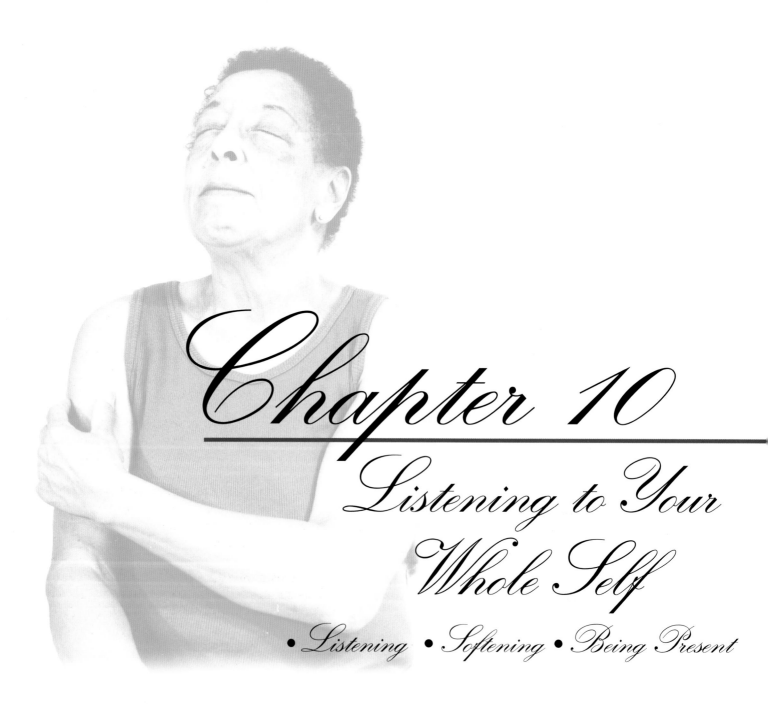

Chapter 10

Listening to Your Whole Self

• Listening • Softening • Being Present

LISTENING

Listening is a patient art. Hearing your body's messages requires that you be fully present, desire to hear the message, and have the skill to interpret subtle sensations. The physical messages come from two sources. First, your hands and fingers will learn to feel the level of tension or relaxation in each muscle. At the same time, you will hear messages from your receiving body. Your muscles will feel the sensations from the massage, and either soften and enjoy it or get tighter and resist the touch. Then comes the dance between your hands and your muscles, the conversation between them that directs your touch in ways that bring comfort, softening, and healing. Each will listen and send messages simultaneously. This is the joy and the challenge in self-massage. The body's sensations awaken memories and emotions that are living in the muscles. These become messages to the hands along with the physical communications, and soon thoughts and emotions are being ministered to also. The gifts your body receives are returned to the whole of you, calming and healing each level of your being.

ow in touch are you with different sensations of your body? Are you focused primarily on what you want your body to do for you to the exclusion of being aware of what it wants and needs? Do you notice discomforts early before they become intense pain? Are you aware of the parts of your body that feel comfortable or terrific? Do you get pleasure from walking or exercising? Do you ever dance spontaneously?

It takes time and interest to learn how to listen well to your body. Now that you have learned how to do the basic massage strokes, you can turn your attention to what strokes and style each part of your body likes and needs. You will learn to listen to two sets of information.

First, internal sensations of relaxation or tightening in response to different kinds of touch will let you know what kind of strokes, pressure, and degree of focus your muscles want. These may be different in different areas of your body, and can change from time to time. The other physical means of sensing what is going on in your body involves the sensitivity of your hands and fingers. You will learn to tell the difference between tight muscles and relaxed ones and to notice subtle shifts in the muscles that indicate softening or tensing, allowing you to quickly shift the type of touch you use to one that brings more comfort.

An injured or sore area needs a different approach than a comfortable, flexible one. In this chapter you will continue to solidify your grasp of the different strokes, while you turn your attention toward individualizing your massage techniques for different areas and varying states of muscle tension. You will learn how to listen to your body and hear the messages it sends to you. This is actually a life-long process of hearing more and more subtle messages from muscles when they feel great and when they are injured, stiff, or tired.

I've been a massage therapist for fourteen years, and I am still deepening my ability to receive subtle messages from muscles. It's as if my hands and fingers are having a conversation with the muscles they are massaging: "Oh, you're tight right here. Do you feel that tightness? Does this kind of touch help you to release that? No? Well, how about this approach then? Ah! I can feel you soften a bit. I'll let you settle into that for a minute and then come back and see what's happening and whether you can release some more..." This kind of gentle, inviting approach focuses on becoming an ally with the injured part as well as with the body's innate healing ability, rather than trying to force a change from the outside. It depends on deepening your fingers' ability to feel muscle tension. You have a great advantage in sensitizing your fingers to the status of your muscles since you also will be listening from the inside of your body and giving feedback to your fingers through your internal sensations.

As a massage therapist I learned this lesson in treating myself the hard way. I had fibromyalgia, and had chronically painful hands and arms. I applied some of the techniques I use in my practice to my sore arms. It "hurt good" when I did them, and my muscles seemed to respond well at the time of the massage. Unfortunately after a few hours my arms hurt at least as much as before I worked on them, and hurt just as much or more the next day. It took me a long time to understand that those muscles wanted a different, much lighter touch, and the deeper pressure caused a flare up of pain. When I finally changed to a softer and gentler touch my arms began to respond and to feel better. It was a great lesson to me to listen to my body wisdom rather than to use my "expert knowledge" in deciding how to approach my muscles. I realized that I had bought into our culture's notion of no pain—no gain, even though I am careful with clients to work gently and to invite the body to find softer, more relaxed ways of being.

Most of us assume that a strong massage must be more beneficial than a gentle one. Unfortunately a muscle responds to pain by tightening against it, making it harder for the muscle to receive the healing touch. It may finally let go, but only when it fatigues and can't hang on anymore. Gentler, subtler approaches are more effective in helping the body to release extra tightness. This is one of the most important lessons you can learn from this book; to trust your body wisdom to guide your own massage. It takes time to learn to hear your body's subtle messages, especially when you are still mastering the massage stroke techniques. Be sure to tune into what your body is saying both at the time of the massage and a few hours and a day later in order to receive the full message. If you are just as sore the next day, try another approach.*

The kind of listening you will be doing is like the attitude you assume when you are focusing on a faint or distant sound, a listening pose where your eyes focus off into the distance as you put your whole attention on the subtle sound you are so intent on hearing.

Each of you has a unique body, and it is helpful to learn what your own muscles feel like. Normal, relaxed muscles feel different in different people. Some people have long, flexible muscles; others have shorter and denser ones. Some have dense tissue overlying tight muscles, especially in the neck and shoulders, which make it harder to feel what's happening in the muscles. This is a protective layer the body creates to guard the sore muscles, or may reflect a protective posture toward the world. Approach whatever you notice in your body and muscles without judgment. There are good reasons for them being just as they are. Simply learn about them by listening with your fingers and hands. Almost every person in our culture holds tension in the neck and shoulders; I have only massaged three people out of hundreds that had no tension there. Several exercises throughout the book focus on this part of the body, but you can take a few minutes right now to learn more about how your muscles feel when they are tight and when they are relaxed.

Rub the pads of your fingertips over the muscles where your neck and shoulder join, noticing what they feel like to your fingers. Rock your fingers over these muscles as they extend out over the top of your shoulder, and then feel the muscles that go up your neck. You probably feel some knots or lumps, or ropey muscles. This lets you know what your tight muscles feel like to your fingers. If your tissue is too dense to feel the muscles, don't worry; it will soften as you massage them more. Now think of an area of your body that feels pretty relaxed to you, and do the same kind of exploration with your fingers. Notice how these feel different to your fingers from the tight muscles. This gives you a quick sense of how your own muscles feel in a couple of different states. Exercise 10a explores listening while massaging in more depth.

Our bodies also speak to us as we move. Moving in a very slow and attentive way will give you more information about where your body moves easily and where there are restrictions. Fast movements will slide by these constraints and you may not notice them. Exercise 10b guides you in slow motion self-exploration.

Now you are ready to go deeper into listening to how your body gives you its messages. Relax as you do the exercises and enjoy yourself as you explore the listening aspect of self-massage.

---

* Note: Professional massage therapists are trained in therapies to treat injuries and long-held restrictions. When you receive a professional massage you may experience soreness the day following the massage. As long as the soreness leaves and you feel better after that, this can be a natural outcome of professional therapeutic massage. In self-massage, however, you should avoid causing yourself any pain or soreness.

LISTENING WHILE MASSAGING

Exercise 10a

Introduction

This exercise shifts the focus of your attention to inside your muscles. Let them tell you what kind of stroke to use, how hard to press, and how quickly or slowly to move.

Preparation

Set aside half an hour and gather oil if you want to use it, or wear comfortable clothes. Have your journal and pen next to you. Create the environment you want, with quiet music or stillness, muting the light, and turning off the phone. Do whatever helps you know you are entering a time to give yourself kind, focused attention.

Settle into a comfortable position in the area you've prepared for yourself and begin to turn your focus inward, allowing your eyes to close or to have a soft downward gaze.

Take eight slow, deep breaths, using them to bring yourself fully present. Use the first two to replace tension in your body with softness throughout. With the next two breaths allow your mind to quiet and focus only on being present right now. Let the next two breaths open your heart, feeling the warm light of the love in your heart filling your whole being. With the next two breaths expand your awareness of your soul and your connection with Spirit, sensing the wisdom, love, and healing within and around you.

Let yourself feel grounded as if you had roots that extend down into the nourishing soil. With a sense of peace and comfort, begin the exercise.

DIRECTIONS

1. **Choose one area of your body to focus on, perhaps a hand or arm, or an area that is uncomfortable.**
2. **Begin massaging with gliding, then with kneading, to warm and soften the muscles.**
3. **Follow the messages you hear from your muscles to guide your movements with the strokes you choose to use. Keep your attention on and below the skin and in your muscles.**
4. **Explore each part of this area with kind touch.**
5. **If you notice an increase in warmth and softness inside your muscles, continue with the strokes you are using.**
6. **If your muscles begin to feel tighter or more uncomfortable, adjust your touch to find an approach that softens them into more comfort.**
7. **Notice how this feels to the hand and fingers giving the massage.**
8. **Continue until your muscles feel satisfied with the massage.**

Journal

Write about your experience.

- Note what you learned about that part of your body.
- Which stroke(s) did it like best? How much pressure did it want? Did this change from the beginning to the end?
- What did you learn about how to listen and hear messages from your muscles? Did your thoughts interfere with hearing your muscles' messages?
- Draw a picture of how that part of your body felt before and after your massage.

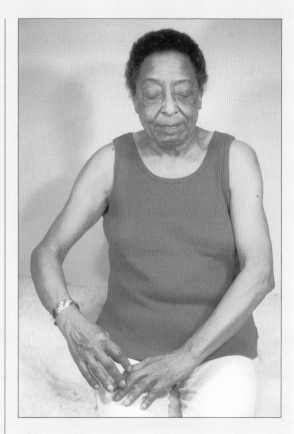

This Week

- Spend a few minutes each day massaging one area of your body, chosen for pleasure or to help with discomfort. Practice listening both from inside your muscles and with your fingers.
- Record your experiences in your journal.

LISTENING THROUGH MOVEMENT
SLOW MOTION

Exercise 10b

Introduction

This exercise is not a goal-oriented one in terms of "getting those muscles stretched." Instead, it uses conscious slow stretching and moving as a powerful way of becoming more and more aware of your body/your self and of discovering how your own body likes to move. Listen to your body as it moves.

Preparation

Prepare a comfortable place, wear comfortable clothing, and have your journal handy. Settle into a comfortable position and begin to turn your focus inward, allowing your eyes to close or to have a soft downward gaze.

Take eight slow, deep breaths, using them to bring yourself fully present. Use the first two to replace tension in your body with softness throughout. With the next two breaths allow your mind to quiet and focus only on being present right now. Let the next two breaths open your heart, feeling the warm light of the love in your heart filling your whole being. With the next two breaths expand your awareness of your soul and your connection with Spirit, sensing the wisdom, love, and healing within and around you.

Let yourself feel grounded as if you had roots that extend down into the nourishing soil. With a sense of peace and comfort, begin the exercise.

DIRECTIONS

1. **Begin with one thumb, and let it lead its own slooooww motion dance. The extreme slowness helps you to "hear" (see, feel) any jerkiness in the movement. The same slow motions will help to heal those restrictions. Fully explore all the directions and shapes your thumb wants to investigate.**

2. **Let your fingers and whole hand join the extremely slow motion.**
3. **Allow your hand and wrist to lead the directions of moving in all the ways they want to explore.**
4. **Let your forearm and elbow join in and then lead.**
5. **Finally, begin the (still very slow) motion of your arm and hand starting from your shoulder.**

Journal

Write about your experience

- What did you discover?
- Where was your movement smooth and where was it jerky?
- Were there directions of movement that were uncomfortable? Did you listen to these messages and stop going in that direction?
- Which movements brought pleasure and comfort?
- What did you discover about the relationships between your thumb, hand, arm, and shoulder?
- Will this help you listen to your body better?

This Week

- Each day revisit this type of listening movement for the same or different parts of your body.
- When you repeat this exercise for the same area, notice the changes you experience in the amount of stiffness, jerkiness, and comfort.
- Continue listening to the Self-Blessing exercise each day.
- Record your experiences in your journal.

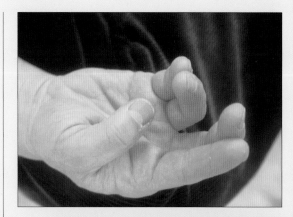
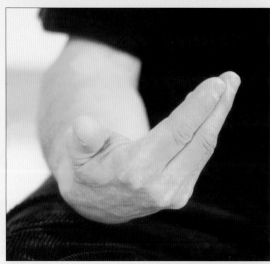
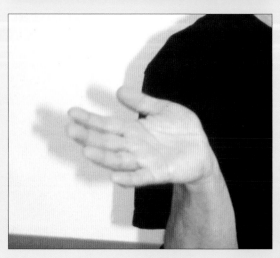

SOFTENING

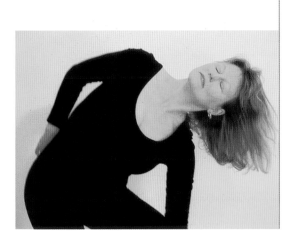

ou now have a sense of listening to your body's messages. Now we will build on that and deepen your ability to connect with your body through moving toward softening and releasing. Many of us move through our days holding our bodies with tension. You may do this and not be aware of it. If you are holding your body tightly, restraining your emotions and feelings, or pulling back on your creative expression, these restrictions will affect you on every level of your being. In our fast-paced world almost all of us feel the effects of stress and strain on our bodies; neck and shoulder tension is endemic in Western culture.

As you learn to listen more closely to your body, you will begin to notice how your body responds in different situations; when your body rests easily and when and where it stiffens. Inherent in the process of softening your body is releasing areas that hold chronic tension or tightness. This sounds simple, but you may come up against powerful holding patterns and restrictions.

Most of us have developed protective habits over our lives, often as children. Body holding patterns always are formed as a protection against a threat, whether it was a physical threat (e.g., to guard an area after an injury) or an emotional or mental threat (e.g., tightness in the chest or throat to hold in words that were unacceptable to parents, or whole body guarding to protect against external aggression). Unfortunately, after forming such restrictions, the body does not go back to check whether they are still needed. After the injury has healed or the threat is gone, the muscle no longer needs to guard itself; yet the body still holds the pattern. We must consciously revisit the tightness in order to release it.

Massage therapists address such patterns in most clients, but you can also do a great deal to release old habits of tension with self-massage. It takes attention and patience with your body, somewhat similar to helping a child learn something they think they cannot do. Your body understands the language of touch with kind presence. Old tight patterns will gradually shift. Since emotions are tied up in these bodily restrictions, be prepared to support yourself in case they come up. You may want to share some of these experiences with an understanding friend; and recording them in your journal will help you deepen the release.

Be sure to shift your framework and attitudes when you begin this practice. You need to approach your body with compassion, not with judgment; with self-acceptance, not rejection; with an open heart, not a closed mind. This may be an unaccustomed state for you. If so, be patient as you practice these exercises; you will soon be able to include the parts of yourself that you now may want to reject. Learn to treat yourself with the same love and acceptance you would give a beloved child or lover or friend. As you expand your ability to be kinder to yourself, you may find greater abilities to be open and loving with others in your life.

You may also find yourself moving more spontaneously and enjoying your body in motion. Our bodies like to move, no matter what kind of restrictions they may have. Restrictions merely change the degree of the motions, not the body's innate pleasure to move. We forget how regenerating movement can be, especially when it comes naturally from inside.

The next two exercises in this chapter focus on softening your attitudes and thoughts into greater self-acceptance and enjoyment of who you are, moving away from any societal messages you have internalized about how you should look or be. The third exercise builds on the previous movement exercises to bring creativity and play into the process of softening.

AFFIRMATIONS
"I SOFTEN"

Exercise 10c

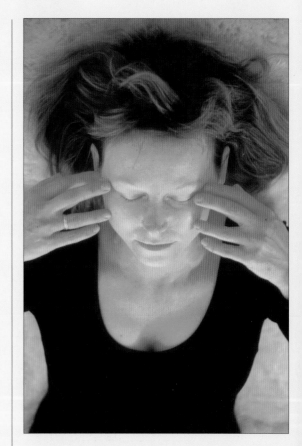

Introduction

Speaking or writing "I soften" is a potent mantra or affirmation. Learning to soften your body, mind, and emotions brings you powerfully closer to realizing your wholeness. When you do this exercise focus on the different aspects you may want to soften, including your relationships and the roles you play in the world. Physically, be aware of muscle or stomach tension, of headaches triggered by stress, or other ways stress emerges for you. Mentally, you may want to soften preoccupying trains of thought, or an inner critical voice, or judgments of others. Emotionally, be aware of restricting emotions, or long-held resentments, anger, or guilt; acknowledge your own unique demons. Notice patterns of tightness in all areas of yourself and your life that limit the free-flow of energy. Notice what keeps you from feeling a full sense of your soul and your connection with Spirit. Give yourself enough time with each section in this exercise to allow your inner wisdom to offer spontaneous insights that you wouldn't have thought with your active mind.

Preparation

Gather your journal and pen and settle into a comfortable place.

DIRECTIONS

1. Take five or ten minutes now and each day this week to write a list of phrases that begin with "I soften."
2. Begin and end with five or six repetitions of "I soften," and invite your body to let go as you repeat the phrase.
3. Include these types of openers for your phrases.
   • I soften...
   • I soften into...
   • I soften my...
   • I soften so that...
   • I soften around...
4. Notice where you are first aware of softening—in your body, your thoughts, your emotions, or your soul. Then invite and notice how this relaxing expands to include the rest of you.
5. Place your hands over any area that would like the physical support for softening.
6. Write a note about what you have discovered from this process.

This Week

- Repeat this exercise each day.
- Record in your journal what you discover about your tensions and softening.
- Where do you carry your tension? Answer this question for your body, your thoughts, your emotions, and your relationship to your soul and to Spirit.
- What have you discovered about the effects of softening for you?

LOOKING WITH KIND EYES
RELEASING JUDGMENTS #1; MIRROR EXERCISE #2

Exercise 10d

Introduction

Faces are so important. They are the main way we recognize each other. Our faces express our love, compassion, fear, or anger. Unfortunately, in our culture many people focus on what they feel is "wrong" about their faces, judging themselves on superficial qualities. I invite you to try another approach. Take a few minutes to look at your face with kinder eyes, looking for something deeper than the surface. Try looking at "flaws" in your facial appearance as the things that make your face unique and recognizable as you and nobody else.

Preparation

Gather your journal and pen, and place a mirror where you can easily see your face.

Settle into a comfortable position in the area you've prepared for yourself and begin to turn your focus inward, allowing your eyes to close or to have a soft downward gaze.

Take eight slow, deep breaths, using them to bring yourself fully present. Use the first two to replace tension in your body with softness throughout. With the next two breaths allow your mind to quiet and focus only on being present right now. Let the next two breaths open your heart, feeling the warm light of the love in your heart filling your whole being. With the next two breaths expand your awareness of your soul and your connection with Spirit, sensing the wisdom, love, and healing within and around you.

Let yourself feel grounded as if you had roots that extend down into the nourishing soil. With a sense of peace and comfort, begin the exercise.

DIRECTIONS

1. Review your journal notes for Exercise 2b: Seeing Softness where you jotted down all the thoughts you had about your face before and after you did the Self-Blessing.
2. Look at your face and notice if there are any changes in how you see yourself since you began doing the Self-Blessing regularly and giving yourself KindTouch.
3. Look at your surface appearance and notice what you've thought of as "flaws," and then let your attention come from your kind heart, and allow yourself to accept and love all of your face, your unique appearance.
4. Focus on gratitude for all that your face brings to you—taste, smell, touch, sight, and expression of your feelings. See any wrinkles as memories of your laughter and diverse experiences that make up your life.
5. Give your face some kind touch with your eyes closed.
6. Open your eyes and notice if your response to your face in the mirror changes.

Journal

Write about your experience.

- Record in your journal what you discover about your tensions and softening.
- Where do you carry your tension? Answer this question for your body, your thoughts, your emotions, and your relationship to your soul and to Spirit.
- What have you discovered about the effects of softening for you?

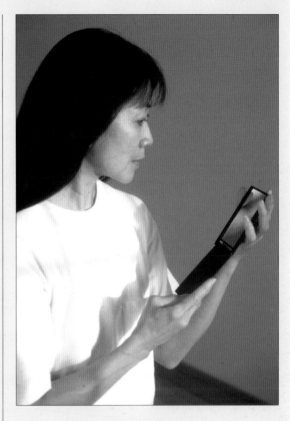

This Week

- Repeat this exercise each day.
- Practice letting your face be the entryway for feelings of affection for your inner self, looking for the things that remind you of your true self.
- Notice how your face softens as you change how you approach it.

TURN STRETCHING
INTO A DANCE

Exercise 10e

Introduction

Give yourself private space to explore your body's language of movement. By softening into the ways your body loves to move, you can become free to express yourself through your body. You have already done some stretching and explored some slow movement with your hand, arm, and shoulder in Exercise 10b. This exercise asks you to take this one step further, moving into dance and play. It can be a great challenge and also a joy to be present without judgment while you move and dance. Take this lightly and enjoy yourself!

Preparation

Arrange a private space with room to move without interruptions.

Take eight slow, deep breaths, using them to bring yourself fully present. Use the first two to replace tension in your body with softness throughout. With the next two breaths allow your mind to quiet and focus only on being present right now. Let the next two breaths open your heart, feeling the warm light of the love in your heart filling your whole being. With the next two breaths expand your awareness of your soul and your connection with Spirit, sensing the wisdom, love, and healing within and around you.

Let yourself feel grounded as if you had roots that extend down into the nourishing soil. With a sense of peace and comfort, begin the exercise.

DIRECTIONS

1. Review your journal entries for Exercise 10b: Listening Through Movement, and remember what you enjoyed most.
2. Begin by stretching your arms and hands first, then gradually add more parts of your body until your whole

body is involved in stretching. Fully experience your movements and inner sensations.
3. Now, tune into your body intuition and turn the stretching into a sinuous dance of your arms and hands, head and neck, legs and feet, and torso. Begin with one arm or with your whole body. Just let your body find its own pleasure in motion.
4. When you feel warmed up, let your body play in whatever way it wants.

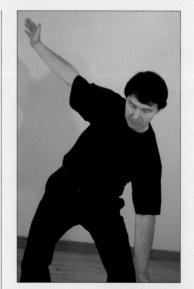

Journal

Write about your experience.

- What did you discover about how your body likes to move?
- How fully were you able to immerse yourself in this experience?
- Did you have judging thoughts? If you did, were you able to let them go and become present again?

This Week

- Turn stretching into a dance for even a few minutes every day.
- Let your body move with more spontaneity with every activity throughout the day. Begin to experience yourself as dancing through your life.
- Note your discoveries and changes in your journal.

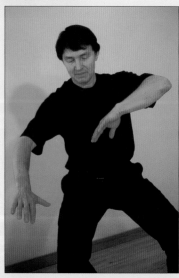

Follow your own pacing and comfort; keep the movements slow and luxurious or allow your body to move faster, as long as you follow your body's pleasure growing out of this stretching dance. If you find that some of your motions cause discomfort, pull back on that gesture and begin again, exploring within your envelope of comfort. It doesn't require large or fast movements for your body to be able to express itself. Balance your motions with your body's abilities, flexibility, limitations, and comfort level. Resist any impulses to observe yourself or to judge whether you're doing it "right." There is no right, there is only following your body's pleasure in movement. It will look different for each of you.

BEING PRESENT

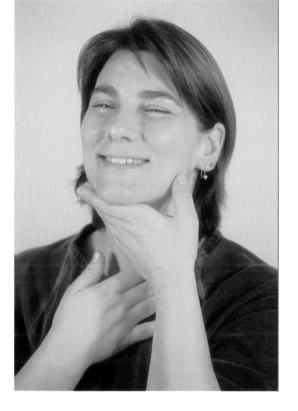

hen we are present we are alive to ourselves and to all that is around us in the moment. Mindfulness meditation, popularized by Jon Kabot-Zinn, focuses on simply being in the moment, being aware. In our result-oriented and stimulation-dependent culture it takes intention to find time to simply be.

You have already spent time listening to your body, bringing more softness into your muscles, and releasing some judgments you may have had about yourself. Now we will focus on the power of presence to deepen your healing path.

Being present for yourself includes being open to areas of both comfort and discomfort. Each of you may find it easier to connect with one than the other. Many people are out of touch with their bodies enough that the only sensation they feel is pain when it gets to the level that it breaks through their awareness. Take a minute to think about how sensitive you are to your body's more subtle messages. Are you as aware of where your body is comfortable and happy as you are of the places that hurt or feel stiff? How big must a pain become before you pay attention to it? Are you aware of subtle messages of discomfort before they become larger?

If your knee hurts, you may disconnect from yourself in two ways. First, you may split off from the sore knee. The second separation is wider ranging. Often the pain and your resistance to it can distract you from noticing the other, larger areas of your body that feel fine. Comfort and pain each offer their own challenges to being present. We must be able to simply be with them, not asking for a change, but simply experiencing comfort and being present with compassion for pain or illness. This is difficult to do, to be unattached to wanting more of the one, and much less of the other.

The next exercise will focus on being present with areas of comfort. You may find that there are vast areas of comfort inside you of which you are totally unaware. The second exercise will give you an opportunity to be present with an area in your body that is not comfortable. It may be painful, stiff, nauseated, full of fatigue, or whatever is true for you.

Being present does not ask anything of you except to experience "what is." Treat each exercise like a meditation—when thoughts come into your head, simply turn your attention back to the experience you are focusing on. Have no judgment about whatever thoughts arise. Simply return to your focus.

You cannot move away from 'now.' Whatever you do, however fast you run; you will be in the now.

Osho

EXPLORING COMFORT

Exercise 10f

Introduction

This exercise increases your ability to experience those areas in you that are comfortable and relaxed so that you can enjoy your body and life more. If you find you are unable to tune into comfort because your pain is too distracting, do Exercise 10g first, and then return to this one.

Preparation

Settle into a comfortable position in the area you've prepared for yourself and begin to turn your focus inward, allowing your eyes to close or to have a soft downward gaze.

Take eight slow, deep breaths, using them to bring yourself fully present. Use the first two to replace tension in your body with softness throughout. With the next two breaths allow your mind to quiet and focus only on being present right now. Let the next two breaths open your heart, feeling the warm light of the love in your heart filling your whole being. With the next two breaths expand your awareness of your soul and your connection with Spirit, sensing the wisdom, love, and healing within and around you.

Let yourself feel grounded as if you had roots that extend down into the nourishing soil. With a sense of peace and comfort, begin the exercise.

DIRECTIONS

1. **Take a moment to be aware of each part of you that is stiff, sore, or painful; and wrap each one in an imaginary blanket of kindness so they can rest there while you focus on other areas.**
2. **Bring your awareness to the areas of your body that are comfortable and easy. Even if there is only one small area, you will be able to find it with**

patience. Place your hands or your attention there.

3. **Take a few minutes to notice the subtleties of these good feelings of relaxation and ease and invite them to grow and expand. Is there a sense of warmth? Softening? An indescribable but recognizable feeling you know means comfort or relaxation? Does the comfort expand? In what ways?**
4. **Ask each area of focus the questions below and simply wait for an answer to appear.**
   - **What do you want to say to me?**
   - **What do you need from me?**
   The response could be in words, physical shifts, or simply knowing what the message is. If none appears, simply move on. We will spend time with other ways to talk to your body later.
5. **What do you want to say to this area of your body?**
6. **Express your gratitude for the comfort and pleasure it gives you.**

Journal

Write about your experience.

- Was it difficult to notice where you are comfortable?
- How do you experience relaxed comfort in your body?
- What happened when you invited your sense of comfort to expand?
- What messages did your comfort have for you? What did you say to it?
- Compare the size of your areas of comfort before and after the exercise.
- Draw a picture of your body, showing areas of pain and of ease. You can draw two if you want, one from before this exercise and one after it.

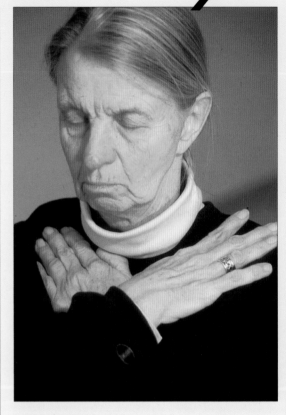

This Week

- Each day spend some time noticing where in your body you feel easy and comfortable. Let those sensations grow.
- This week practice presence in simple things you do. For example, every time (or at least once a day) you eat or drink anything, bring your whole attention to your experience of it. Notice how the food or liquid feels as it is in your mouth and as it goes down to your stomach. Notice if you feel anything else on a physical or energetic level.
- Note in your journal if and how it becomes easier to become aware of your comfort. Does this affect your painful areas?

EXPLORING DISCOMFORT
RELEASING JUDGMENTS #2

Exercise 10g

Introduction

This exercise focuses on increasing your ability to simply be present with areas of pain. You will be using your mind as well as your body and emotions. Hold all of these areas in the gentle hands of your soul, and beyond that let yourself be aware of Spirit holding all of you. You may find that some of the stiffness or pain softens a bit, or it may stay the same while being held in a container of peace and comfort. Our ability to hold our pain with loving hands reduces the suffering connected to our pain.

Preparation

Have your journal and pen handy.

DIRECTIONS

1. Choose an area of your body that is uncomfortable, or that you don't like, or that you resent or ignore.
2. Put your feelings or attitudes toward this area into words in your journal. Identify what you don't like about it.
3. Take eight slow, deep breaths, using them to bring yourself fully present. Use the first two to replace tension in your body with softness throughout. With the next two breaths allow your mind to quiet and focus only on being present right now. Let the next two breaths open your heart, feeling the warm light of the love in your heart filling your whole being. With the next two breaths expand your awareness of your soul and your connection with Spirit, sensing the wisdom, love, and healing within and around you. Let yourself feel grounded as if you had roots that extend down into the nourishing soil.
4. Connect to your inner wisdom and the love and compassion available there.
5. Look again at the rejected or painful place in your body from the position of compassion, and rest your hands or attention on this area.
6. Notice what you feel or sense in this area.
7. Notice if your pain or your attitude changes as a result of your kind attention. Let the area of pain know that whether it changes or not, you will be there to support it.
8. Ask this area these questions and simply wait for an answer to appear.
   • What do you want to say to me?
   • What do you need from me?
9. What do you want to say to this area?
10. Express your gratitude for the messages you have received.

Journal

Write about your experience.

- Was it difficult to bring a kind focus to the area you chose?
- What happened when you rested your kind attention to this area...in your body and in your thoughts and feelings?
- What messages did it have for you? What does it need from you?
- What did you say to it?
- Is there a difference in the amount or kind of pain and suffering you experience after this exercise?
- Draw a picture of what this part of your body feels like. If it changed, draw before and after pictures.

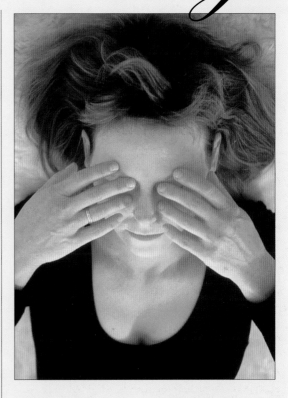

This Week

- Bring your awareness to a painful part of your body each day and offer it compassion and companionship. Notice if it changes gradually as it receives this kind of attention, or if your relationship to it changes. As you become more used to relating in a kinder manner to forgotten parts of your body, expand this attention to other areas as well.
- Record your experiences and learning in your journal.

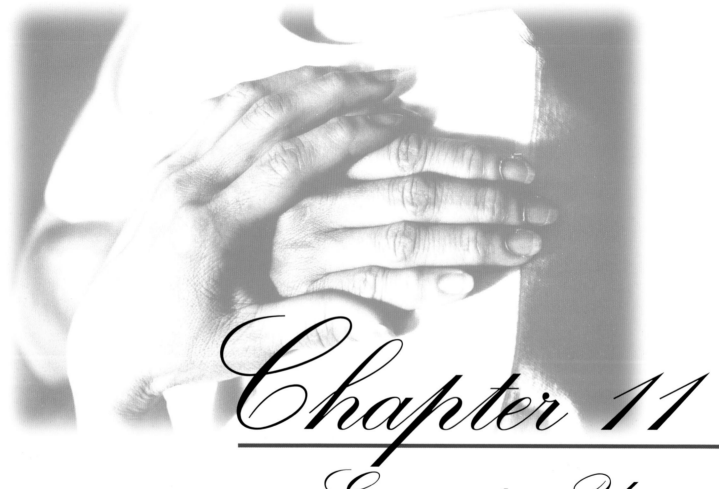

Chapter 11

Expanding Your Experience of Wholeness

• Giving & Receiving • Balancing • Loving & Forgiving

When one person gives a massage to another, there is an identified "giver" and "receiver." Even in this situation, where the roles seem to be so clearly defined, they can blur in a heart-felt interchange. Something is set in motion that is a two-way experience; the giver receives and the receiver gives. Both people come away from the massage feeling relaxed, peaceful, and connected.

When rubbing a sore spot on your body, you probably don't pay attention to your two roles—giving and receiving; you simply try to make yourself feel better. It is a challenge to become aware of the qualities of each of these roles while massaging yourself and, eventually, learn to hold them both in your awareness simultaneously. Self-massage offers a great way to learn to experience yourself as both giver-and-receiver in all aspects of your life—eating good food, bathing and caring for your body, choosing what to wear, spending time with friends, working, making a home, and so forth. You will begin to recognize how you can bring KindTouch to yourself in everything you do.

There are other ways we give and receive within ourselves. Our bodies can help us to release uncomfortable thoughts and emotions. I have a critical voice that tells me I have not done things well enough. I hadn't paid that much attention to it because it was just a part of my background noise; but one day after doing the Self-Blessing (Exercise 2a) every morning for a while, I noticed that it was my body that reacted when I was criticizing myself. I became aware of physical discomfort and heard my body telling me in essence, "I don't like that. Please don't say that!" Then I would think to hold my hand over my heart or stroke my hand over my chest as a way to calm and quiet myself. It helped me change that negative attitude. By calming my body, I could then let that calmness come back into the rest of me, and the critical voice was replaced by self-acceptance

and more peace. As you choose kindness over self-criticism, you actually ground your soul's loving wisdom in your body, and then extend it to your heart and mind.

Once we experience abstract concepts or feelings in our bodies (like releasing negativity or bringing forgiveness and love to ourselves), we have a physically grounded knowledge of those feelings. We can access those emotions more easily through our body memory, rather than just wishing we felt happy instead of depressed. We begin to take action to move toward a desired state of mind and being.

Experiencing ourselves as givers and receivers simultaneously as a means of feeling our wholeness may seem like an abstract concept. Yet, when we can identify these roles through our relationship to our bodies, self-massage becomes a natural path to experiencing wholeness. Our hearts, minds, and souls are working through our hands to give kind touch, and our bodies receive it. And slowly, as our bodies become accustomed to this gift of kindness, they remind us when we return to old negative habits. Every part of ourselves becomes present and involved in the process, eventually giving us the concrete experience of ourselves as whole.

Each of us is a whole person; we are Spirit and matter, inextricably linked. We are not even body and mind, emotions and soul, as if there were separate parts of ourselves that we combine in some way when thinking about ourselves. The totality of who we are is much more than the sum of the parts. Words are powerful, and we tend to forget that we are indivisible when we talk about something happening to our bodies or to our minds. Anything that happens in us or to us happens on every level, not just to the part we identify as affected. For example, a major loss affects more than our emotions; it affects our bodies (witness the increased death rate in people whose spouse died within the last year) and minds (remember your preoccupation and inability to concentrate after a major loss) and our souls (a major loss can shake or strengthen a person's faith in Spirit). The same thing happens with a physical illness or injury; every part of a person is affected. Since we are indivisible, every thought, feeling, sensation, and belief impacts every other part of ourselves.

> *In you, as in every embodied being, the earth and the sky are meeting: it is a love affair of earth and sky.*
>
> Osho

GIVING AND RECEIVING
MASSAGE FOR NECK AND SHOULDERS

Exercise 11a

Introduction

This exercise focuses on massaging tense neck and shoulders, inviting you to move back and forth between being aware of yourself as giver and as receiver. Then, if you can sense both at once, you will begin to have a direct experience of wholeness. Your wholeness here includes your loving heart, the wisdom of your mind, and the transcendence of your soul, along with your receiving body. More than the techniques you use, the state you create within yourself generates the healing touch that comes through in the massage.

Preparation

Gather oil and/or comfortable clothing. If you use oil, keep the room warm so you don't get chilled. Settle into a comfortable position in the area you've prepared for yourself and begin to turn your focus inward, allowing your eyes to close or to have a soft downward gaze.

Take eight slow, deep breaths, using them to bring yourself fully present. Use the first two to replace tension in your body with softness throughout. With the next two breaths allow your mind to quiet and focus only on being present right now. Let the next two breaths open your heart, feeling the warm light of the love in your heart filling your whole being. With the next two breaths expand your awareness of your soul and your connection with Spirit, sensing the wisdom, love, and healing within and around you.

Let yourself feel grounded as if you had roots that extend down into the nourishing soil. With a sense of peace and comfort, begin the exercise.

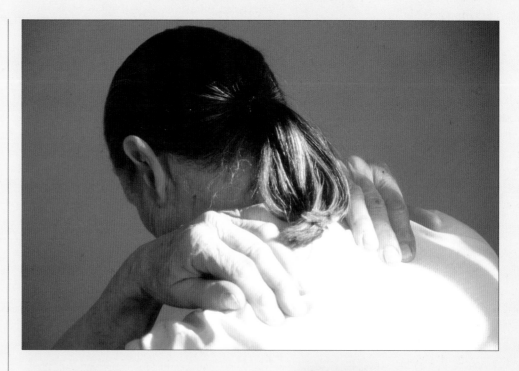

DIRECTIONS

1. Refer back to your journal notes from *Exercise 10a: Listening While Massaging* for reminders about favorite strokes and how you were able to listen to your body's messages.
2. Either sit up or lie on your back or on one side. Lying down allows the muscles to relax more completely.
3. Place your attention on your neck and shoulders. How do they feel right now?
4. Let them know you will bring the kind of touch they want, and ask them to let you know just what they want in each moment, as their needs change. Notice if there is a shift in your neck and shoulders merely from focusing in this way.

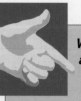

When lying on your side, use a pillow that keeps your neck aligned with your spine. When lying on your back, either use no pillow or place one only under your head, so your hands can reach under your neck.

5. Rest one hand on your opposite shoulder—if you are lying on your back you can do both shoulders with each hand on the same-side shoulder. Notice if the sensations in your shoulder(s) shift after a minute of this kind attention through holding.
6. Begin massaging by gliding across your neck and shoulder in either direction, and then do some gentle kneading to warm and soften the muscles.

7. Let your intuition and the shifting sensations in your muscles guide your strokes and touch, whether they want soothing or more focused pressure.

8. Let your attention move back and forth between your receiving body and your giving hands, heart, mind, and soul.

9. Repeat steps 5-8 with your other shoulder.

10. When you feel complete, bring your attention back to the place where you are resting.

Journal

Write about your experience in your journal.

- Was it easier to get in touch with yourself as giver or as receiver?
- How was it to connect with the role less easily accessed?
- What was your experience of moving your focus back and forth between giving and receiving?
- Did you experience a blend of giving and receiving in every level of your being–body, mind, heart, and soul?
- What did you learn about yourself?

This Week

- Each day take some time to massage one area of your body and focus on being aware of both giving and receiving.
- Move toward becoming more adept at feeling giving and receiving simultaneously, increasing your ability to experience your wholeness.
- Note any changes in your experience in your journal.

Remember to deepen your awareness before deepening into more pressure

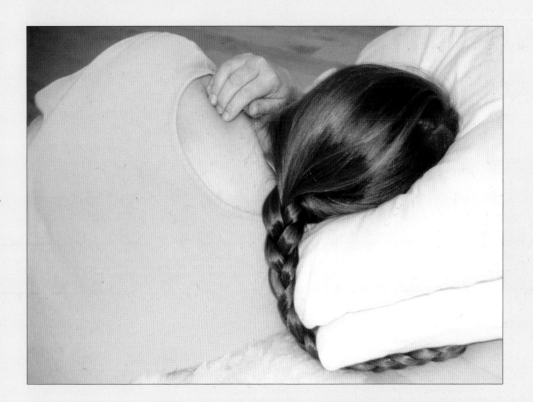

The gentlest thing in the world overcomes the hardest thing in the world. That which has no substance enters where there is no space

Tao Te Ching

Chapter 11 – *Expanding Your Experience of Wholeness*

*D*o you feel you have good balance in your life? For most of us balance is an area where we struggle. With our focus on producing more and more, and taking on many roles in our lives, we are just racing to get everything done. We say we will stop and get balanced after we complete our next big project, but then we always replace the last one with another until we don't know how to jump off the train, and we keep racing down the tracks.

I used to believe that I could figure out the secret to balancing my life, and once I had found the key, I would use it to get my life balanced, and there I would remain, once and for all, balanced. I was disappointed at first to learn that it doesn't work that way; but now I am relieved. I no longer judge myself every time I tip out of equilibrium. I pay attention and make corrections sooner, before I get into extreme states of imbalance.

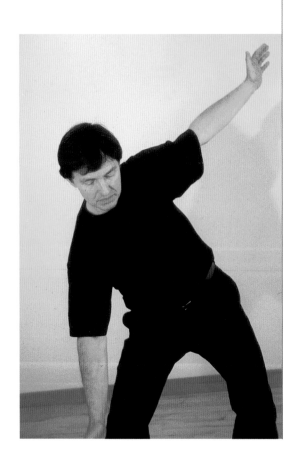

Balance is not a destination, but a way of riding our way through life; it's noticing when we are leaning too far in one direction and then correcting our course to come back toward center. Our bodies do this naturally all the time—regulating our body temperature when it's hot or cold outside; absorbing food, keeping needed nutrients and releasing what's not needed; adjusting our fluid and electrolyte balance when we drink a lot of water (or not enough) or when we exercise hard (or when we don't). Our bodies work to maintain balance from the cellular level to the musculature and everything in between—24 hours a day, 7 days a week.

A lot of areas in our lives need balancing—being and doing, work and play, exercise and rest, time with others and time alone, happiness and sadness, taking in and releasing, contracting and expanding, inhaling and exhaling. Each of us has our own unique list reflecting our experiences and personalities. Each area affects our bodies, either directly or through the repercussions of our emotions.

The balance or imbalance in our lives shows up in our bodies. If we have avoided certain difficult issues in our lives we tend to store them in our bodies. Then eventually the body complains about it with pain in that area. There are some predictable relationships between emotional issues and areas of the body, and others are unique to each of us. Many common connections between physical and psychological conditions are depicted in figures of speech we use—we shoulder our burdens, carry the weight of the world on our backs, find someone a pain in the neck, feel heartsick over the loss of a loved one, or find it hard to stand up for ourselves. Grief often shows up in shoulders and upper backs. As you massage different areas of your body, stay open to flashes of emotion or images that may come and go; these will tell you about emotions you may be storing in certain muscles. In fact some people, who have worked out difficult issues in counseling yet find the depression or anger hanging on, find that a series of bodywork treatments helps to release the lingering feelings. The body stores them and when the muscular holding patterns are released, the left over emotions go with them. Exercises that deal more directly with these kinds of issues will be presented in Chapter 12: Supporting Healing.

Our bodies also get out of balance when we don't recognize sensations of pain or discomfort. When we ignore discomforts, our ability to feel pleasure is also diminished. Unfortunately, if we ignore pain and grow numb to our bodies, the first feelings we notice when we open to our sensations are the strongest ones, so the pain comes back into awareness first. When we persist in staying focused on tuning into and responding to the body's messages with kindness, we gain the benefits of recovering all the pleasurable sensations also. Remember your experience with Exercises 10f and 10g, which focused on being present with comfort as well as discomfort.

John's Story

One of the things about getting older is getting used to the fact that it takes longer to care for myself—my muscles and my whole body, and learning to like taking care of myself. When you are younger you sometimes abuse your body and you can take it; but now I realize I have to take care of it and do things I should have been doing all along. It takes time out of the day. At first I resented the time; I couldn't do other things that I liked to do. I had to walk more, which meant reading less. I couldn't lead as many organizations and I had to learn to think about my body. It isn't automatic anymore. But I have come to like doing these things; I enjoy taking care of my body now. That's the way it is and I like it.

Since most of us know well how to keep busy working, I use the example of balancing work with play here. Many people don't allow themselves to indulge in play. For children, play is vital, not only for feeling alive, but as the means to learn about the world. We encourage them in playful pursuits, and relive our enjoyment of play when we watch them. For many adults playing has lost its legitimacy and they deprive themselves of a vital, natural expression. Before reading on, think about how (and if) you play, and about what it gives you. Does it feed your soul? Does it feel like just another kind of work? Is all of your play competitive? If so, does it bring you what you want in play? Is it quiet? Are you active? Do you prefer to play with others? Or alone? Is there any variety in your play? Do you play but label it something else? One of my friends calls it "wasting time," so while she enjoys it, it is guilty pleasure, with the guilt being the emotion that hangs around the longest.

Play involves you wholeheartedly in something that brings you pleasure, where you lose track of time because of your immersion in it. It leads to re-creation of your life and energy. Julia Cameron, in *The Artist's Way*, speaks about creativity in this same way. It involves every level of yourself and expresses something whole in you, whether you label it play or not. If painting or playing bridge or tennis brings you joy, it's play. If it brings you tension and anxiety because of the competition or the need to perform well, it may not be play for you. Play also is a place to take risks, an important part of life; learn how much risk is the right amount for you. Find what your play is, where you express your creativity, what makes you laugh or excites you; and pursue it! We all need revitalization, spontaneity, and creativity.

You can also be revitalized by approaching all the things you do playfully—by being present in the moment with something you enjoy. Your work can also be your play when understood this way. It's so easy to write those sentences, and it's often such a challenge to do it! Find the things that delight you—they will be unique to you—and include them in a balanced way in your life.

This chapter's exercises invite you to explore balance in your life through physical balance, contemplation, and journaling. Have fun with them!

...the former brawling, gun-collecting fire chief who told me he had 'the inner life of a potato' before healing himself of prostate cancer... had intuitively recognized...that his healing would require, above all, 'a deep kindness.'

Marc Barasch

STANDING IN BALANCE

Exercise 11b

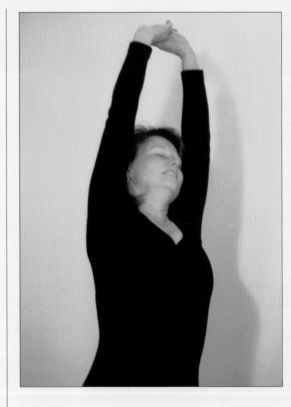

Introduction

Physical balance grounds us and gives us a base from which to respond to unexpected occurrences. As we age, balance becomes less automatic, and deserves our focus and attention. Those without a firm sense of balance in their bodies are more likely to fall and injure themselves. Hip fractures in the elderly lead to an increased risk of death in the next year, as well as less freedom of movement.

DIRECTIONS

1. Stand on one leg and notice whether it is easy or difficult to balance in this position.
2. If it is easy, increase the difficulty—
   • Move your arms or the other leg.
   • Close your eyes while standing still.
   • Move your arms or other leg with your eyes closed.
3. If it continues to be easy, notice how your body feels, and move the rest of your body in a dance while still standing on one leg.
4. Change legs and repeat steps 1-3. You don't need to continue the exercise beyond this point, if it remains easy.
5. If balancing on one leg is difficult, take a minute to stand on both legs and take eight slow, deep breaths.
   • Use the first two to relax your body.
   • Use the second two to quiet your mind and bring your focus inward.
   • With the next set of two breaths open your heart to yourself.
   • In the final two breaths expand your sense of connection to your soul and to Spirit.
6. Place your attention on your feet and focus on your feet meeting the floor or ground firmly. Imagine you have roots or energy that go deep into the earth. Take a minute to imagine how these roots are shaped (a large single root going straight down, or a branching set of roots).
7. Focus your gaze on one spot in front of you, and bring your attention to balance in your body. Keeping your focus on your roots going deeply into the earth, extend your arms out to the sides, shift your weight onto one leg, and slowly lift the other leg.
8. Notice if this manner of focusing makes your balance better.
9. Try adding levels of difficulty while you keep your center focused on your roots and your eyes focused on one spot:
   • Have your arms at your sides
   • Decrease the level of light in the room.
   • Close your eyes.
   • Move a combination of one or two of your arms; then add the other leg.

Note: Don't try this while in the shower; you could slip and fall. Do this exercise only in situations where you can safely catch your balance again.

Increase the level of difficulty as your balance improves.

Keep track of your improvement in your journal.

Journal

Write about your experience.

• What did you discover about your balance?
• Did your balance change when you focused on your roots?

This Week and beyond

• Bring your focus on balance into your daily activities, practicing physical balance while doing your regular routines. Gear this to the level at which your balance first felt challenged. For example, you can practice while standing in line at a store or bank, while drying your feet or putting lotion on them.

PLAYFUL SELF-MASSAGE OR MOVEMENT

Exercise 11c

Introduction

In this exercise you are invited to give yourself a playful self-massage or to move your body in play. Forget any rational thoughts about what will be good for you; simply follow your playful body and have fun.

Preparation

Have your journal and pen or pencil nearby. Wear comfortable clothes or have massage oil handy in a warm room. Assure complete privacy. Settle into a comfortable position in the area you've prepared for yourself and begin to turn your focus inward, allowing your eyes to close or to have a soft downward gaze.

Take eight slow, deep breaths, using them to bring yourself fully present. Use the first two to replace tension in your body with softness throughout. With the next two breaths allow your mind to quiet and focus only on being present right now. Let the next two breaths open your heart, feeling the warm light of the love in your heart filling your whole being. With the next two breaths expand your awareness of your soul and your connection with Spirit, sensing the wisdom, love, and healing within and around you.

Let yourself feel grounded as if you had roots that extend down into the nourishing soil. With a sense of peace and comfort, begin the exercise.

DIRECTIONS

1. Choose whether you would like to play through self-massage or through moving.
2. Listen to some favorite music while you do this exercise if you like.
3. Read all the directions below before you begin the self-massage or playful movement.

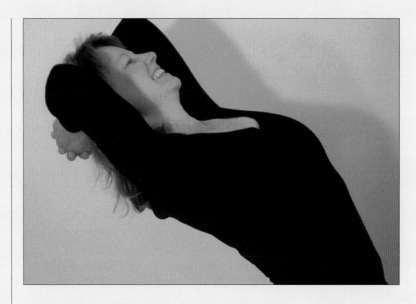

4. Close your eyes and invite your body to lead you. Wait patiently for impulses to emerge; it may have been a long time since you gave your body creative license.
5. Ask your body what sounds fun, and then follow its lead.
6. Let each movement or massage stroke lead into the next one.
7. If you find yourself pausing or hesitating, relax and wait for the next impulse to emerge from within your body, no matter how small the movement or how different it is from the last one.
8. Thank your body for discovering its creativity, even if you feel awkward at first.
9. Revel in your body's sensations. Notice how your body's expression expands to your heart, mind, and soul.
10. If part of you feels uncomfortable, listen and respect that message also. What does your body want to do?
11. Follow your body's lead until you feel complete.

Journal

- Write some frivolous or poetic lines about your experience in your journal.
- Draw shapes or a picture that express what just happened.

This Week

- Each day give yourself a few minutes (or more) to let your body play, either with touch or with movement.
- Note in your journal what you discover about yourself, your body, and play.

Notice the effect of this on how alive you feel.

Notice how you may stop yourself from this kind of play. Just give yourself gentle invitations to continue.

Chapter 11 – Expanding Your Experience of Wholeness

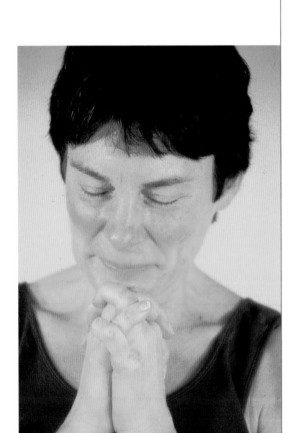

Many of us judge ourselves harshly. If we said the things to others that we say to ourselves we would have few friends, and we might even be guilty of emotional abuse. Take a minute and ask yourself if this applies to you. We criticize our looks, our talents, our attitudes, our habits; and we berate ourselves for any mistakes we make. If most things go well in a day, and one or two things go wrong, which do you focus on? Do you concentrate on the negative and feel bad rather than remembering the more frequent positive things with enjoyment?

It is important to forgive ourselves as well as others, but we often respond superficially to mistakes we make or shortcomings we feel we have, merely by making a quick rationalization or briefly cringing, and moving on. This leaves the underlying self-criticisms unresolved, waiting to catch us the next time. We are so eager to escape our feelings of discomfort that we never fully deal with the self-criticism, which leaves the self-judgment intact and rejects our humanity. When we glance at an error or a blemish and quickly look away, we never give ourselves the time to look at the issue and forgive ourselves (or realize there's nothing to forgive).

A good illustration of such self-judgment comes from one of my clients, Ellen, when she did Exercise 11d, which involves looking at oneself closely in a full-length mirror. She had been aware of some discomfort with changes in her body as she got older, but had not fully acknowledged it. When she took the time to really look at herself she realized she felt disappointed. She said she had always been slim and had never planned on having a middle-aged body, and here she was looking at one. She became aware that up until this point, whenever she caught sight of her body, she had been quickly looking away to avoid seeing what she did not want to see. It was the second part of the exercise (finding gratitude for the gifts her body has given her) that

helped her move past her judgments about her surface appearance. When she met her body from the inside and focused on all it does for her and all it had been through with her, her judgment softened and she was able to connect with herself with love again. She reports that she received a surprising gift over the next few weeks. One day she caught a glimpse of her body in the mirror and heard herself saying, "That's kind of a cute belly." This surprised her, and she was relieved to feel her attitudes changing. She says she does look at her body now instead of turning away, and she feels affection for her constant companion who has been through so much with her. Her desire to be flat-bellied has not completely disappeared, but she is much more accepting of it now.

When another friend heard this story she reacted strongly with anger about the self-doubt our society promotes in older women. She "values the soft rounding of the female body, and equally the strength of being a woman, not a young girl. It's cultural brainwashing that denigrates the fullness of mature female bellies and hips and glamorizes young flat bellies." It takes conscious attention to change culturally instilled beliefs about beauty and values.

When we don't take the time to resolve our self-judgments they remain unseen and unresolved, undermining our self-esteem. A sense of failure combines with all the rest of the criticisms we store (often in our bodies) without being aware of it. We don't understand why we don't feel good about ourselves, and why our bodies feel sluggish. Some people turn the blame on others when things go wrong and stay mad at them instead of healing themselves. Others get depressed or lose all their energy and juice and can't find their natural enthusiasm and interest in any area. Of course, many deaden their sense of failure or emptiness by becoming addicted to alcohol, drugs, eating, sex, or even being a compulsively "nice" person. We use up our creativity by finding self-destructive patterns to distance ourselves from the pain of not feeling loved and accepted enough. If we look for all our needs for love and acceptance to be filled by others, we will continue to be disappointed. It is too big a job for someone else. We must look within ourselves first for this basic need.

Coming to the place of loving our bodies is inextricably linked to the need to forgive our bodies for not living up to our (totally unrealistic) expectations. Our bodily self-rejections appear in several arenas. As you read this, notice if you identify with the ones mentioned here, and see if you have other unique ways of disowning your body. We often judge the parts of ourselves that are not as beautiful as we would like them to be, or areas that we think show some deficiency: blemishes, sags or cellulite; we are too fat or too thin, too short or too tall, too old, too wrinkled, too young or too naive-appearing. We are not very nice when we look upon ourselves.

Giving yourself loving touch conveys forgiveness and acceptance. The other side of this bargain is that you also must receive these gifts. You have had many experiences already with receiving kind touch from yourself; now you have the opportunity to accept some of your most rewarding gifts. Self-massage with the focus of expressing love and forgiveness is very sweet. This chapter concludes with this experience in Exercise 11e.

Martha's Story

I really felt like my back had let me down when I most needed it. I have been mad at my lower back for 10 years now and I'm still not functioning fully. I feel very tender and can't seem to get the whole thing into a place of strength and flexibility. So I have been mad at my back. When I asked my back what it wanted to say to me I first heard this: "I want you to lose weight and stop being so mad at me." That was the beginning but I realized that I was getting a reflection of my own judgment so I waited and softened and listened more deeply and then I heard what I needed to hear: "I have been carrying you through a joyless life until I couldn't do it anymore. I want to move, I love to move, but I can't do it under so much stress." When I heard this I broke down and wept; I have felt myself moving back into that workaholic attitude that I was in when my back first went out. I am working night and day and getting exhausted and doing very little exercise and my back has started to hurt again. I feel enormous gratitude for this message and for my back—I have a built in signal to keep me focused on what really matters.

Why do you want to shut out of your life any uneasiness, any misery, any depression, since after all you don't know what work these conditions are doing inside of you.

Rainer Maria Rilke

SEEING WITH DIFFERENT EYES
WHOLE BODY—
RELEASING JUDGMENTS #3

Exercise 11d

Introduction

It takes courage to face your attitudes about your body, and then change them through forgiveness and gratitude. This exercise gives you the time to see your body and identify the feelings and attitudes you have toward it, and then offers you a way to see it through "different," kinder eyes. Treat yourself kindly and take the time to do it. Facing ourselves squarely can be the hardest thing we do, and can be the most rewarding. You may choose to do this exercise in stages. Each time you come back to it your experience will deepen and your self-acceptance will grow.

Preparation

You'll need an hour of private time, a full-length mirror, a hand mirror, your journal, and favorite pen or pencil. Wear only a robe.

Settle into a comfortable position in the area you've prepared for yourself and begin to turn your focus inward, allowing your eyes to close or to have a soft downward gaze. Take eight slow, deep breaths, using them to bring yourself fully present. Use the first two to replace tension in your body with softness throughout. With the next two breaths allow your mind to quiet and focus only on being present right now. Let the next two breaths open your heart, feeling the warm light of the love in your heart filling your whole being. With the next two breaths expand your awareness of your soul and your connection with Spirit, sensing the wisdom, love, and healing within and around you. Let yourself feel grounded as if you had roots that extend down into the nourishing soil.

With a sense of peace and comfort, begin the exercise.

DIRECTIONS

Read each portion of the instructions, and then take the time to do that part and write about your experience. Approach this with curiosity and a sense of opportunity. If you wish, you can do one section each day. If you do it this way, however, be sure to finish it; the first part can feel discouraging.

Part One: View your whole body

1. Review your journal notes about Exercise 2b: Seeing Softness and Exercise 10d: Looking with Kind Eyes.
2. First, take a minute to look at your face and write down your thoughts and feelings briefly.
3. Then take the time to look at your arms and your hands and see what you notice, what you focus on, what your mind has to say about it, and what feelings come up. Jot these down.
4. Do the same for your legs: the fronts, sides, and backs. Repeat this for your feet. Briefly note down your responses.
5. Now look at your torso: your chest and abdomen, your sides, and use your hand mirror to see your back and buttocks. Jot down your responses.

Part Two: Reflect

1. Now put your robe back on. Write three sentences that summarize your experience so far.
2. Let go of all that has come up. Take eight deep breaths, releasing tension and bringing softness into your body, mind, heart, and soul. Thank yourself for your honesty, and let go of any judgments.
3. Let your curiosity grow about the next part of this experience. Sit down someplace comfortable; perhaps get yourself

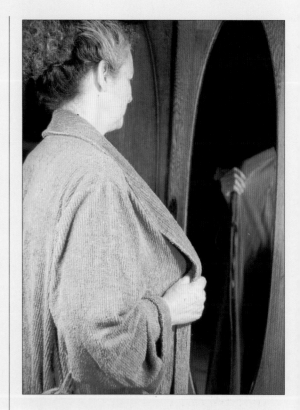

a cup of tea or something that makes you feel at ease.

Part Three: Seeing with new eyes

1. Start with your hands and arms, and think of all they do for you.
   - What do they do that makes your life run smoothly, that gives you pleasure? Consider the things they do that make you feel proud of what you can accomplish and ways they can express compassion and love. Jot these things down in your journal.
   - Allow yourself to experience gratitude for what they do for you; what they have done for you all your life. If there are scars or injuries or disabilities, thank your hands and arms for what they do in spite of the difficulties they may have in doing them.

- Express your gratitude through KindTouch to your hands and arms. Notice what sensations they have when you do this.
- Look at your arms and hands again, with gratitude in your heart, and notice any differences in how you perceive and experience them. Record your responses.

2. Next, turn your attention to your face, head, and neck. The uniqueness of your face allows people to recognize you; it gives expression to your feelings; it is the gateway for important sensations—sight, smell, taste.
    - If your face is lined or wrinkled or has blemishes, think of the number of years you've lived and how those wrinkles reflect those years, and how they reflect your ability to express emotions: to laugh, to smile, to cry, to be in pain, to be angry, to show love and caring.
    - Express your gratitude through KindTouch, and look again at your face with kind eyes.
    - Record your experiences in your journal.

3. Now move your attention to your feet and your legs, and notice how they reflect your life history.
    - What have they done for you? Where have they taken you?
    - Give your gratitude through self-massage and notice any changes in how you see them.
    - Record your responses.

4. Bring your attention to your torso: your chest, abdomen, back, and buttocks.
    - Reflect on how your life is reflected in the shape of your torso.
    - If you are a woman, have you been pregnant? Have you had babies? How does your body reflect this miracle that took place? Have your hormones changed with menopause?
    - If you are a man, how does your body reflect the work you do, the life you lead?

5. Be aware of all the organs inside your torso.
    - Think of how they work effortlessly for you, never ceasing—your heart, lungs, gastro-intestinal system, sexual organs, urinary system, and all your other organs.
    - Remember with gratitude all they have done for you all your life.
    - Use KindTouch to express your gratitude, and look with kind eyes.
    - Record your experiences.

6. Take a minute to focus on your whole body and the miracle it is and all it does for you. Give yourself a blessing. Be thankful if any self-judgments have diminished.

Part Four: Write your experiences in your journal

1. In what ways did your attitudes and feelings change? How much did they change?

2. Did your body look different to you after spending time thinking about your journey with your body and how it has served you? How did it change?

3. How did it feel to forgive your body for its imperfections? Were you able to do this? To what extent?

4. In what ways do you want to continue this journey into compassion, forgiveness, and gratitude for your body and yourself?

This Week
- Each day this week focus again on different parts of your body, giving them your gratitude and forgiveness.
- Look in the mirror at your body each day, getting used to seeing your physical self with kinder eyes.
- Write in your journal about your experiences and growth in this area.

Start a gratitude journal for your body. Every day write five ways you are grateful to your body. If you have trouble thinking of anything, go back to the basics. Remember breathing, seeing, tasting great flavors, hearing beautiful sounds, the ability to walk, to dance, to sing, to speak, to feel textures and sensations, and so on. Make your list unique to you and your own body. Let it lead you to falling in love with your body again.

MASSAGE FOR LOVING AND FORGIVING

Exercise 11e

Introduction

This exercise will give you an opportunity to massage areas of your body about which you have had judgments.

Preparation

Wear comfortable clothes or have massage oil handy, and settle into a comfortable, warm place where you won't be distracted.

Settle into a comfortable position in the area you've prepared for yourself and begin to turn your focus inward, allowing your eyes to close or to have a soft downward gaze. Take eight slow, deep breaths, using them to bring yourself fully present. Use the first two to replace tension in your body with softness throughout. With the next two breaths allow your mind to quiet and focus only on being present right now. Let the next two breaths open your heart, feeling the warm light of the love in your heart filling your whole being. With the next two breaths expand your awareness of your soul and your connection with Spirit, sensing the wisdom, love, and healing within and around you.

Let yourself feel grounded as if you had roots that extend down into the nourishing soil. With a sense of peace and comfort, begin the exercise.

DIRECTIONS

1. **Choose one area of your body that you had a hard time looking at in the mirror, that you ignore or reject, and for which you would like to move toward more acceptance and comfort.**
2. **Focus on curiosity and kindness in approaching this area.**
3. **Remember the first time when you moved away from contact with this part of your body. What was happen-**
ing? Why was it important to distance from that spot at that time?
4. **What has changed so that you want to create a loving and kind relationship with it now?**
5. **Gently place your hand(s) over the area you want to massage with kind touch and let them mold to the shape of your body there. Let the warmth of your hands warm the area. If you cannot reach the spot, do this in your imagination, letting it be as powerful as if you were actually touching it.**
6. **Let your attention rest inside the area from which you have distanced yourself, and take a few minutes to notice what it feels like now. Notice any shifts in sensation within the area as you hold it with loving hands and a curious mind.**
7. **Ask the area what kind of additional touch it wants, and pay attention to your intuition about this. Be open to a variety of possible responses from your body—sensations, words, images, or thoughts appearing in your head that feel true.**
8. **Always begin with gentle gliding over the whole area and gradually increase your focus and depth of touch to help the area receive your touch. Remember not to start with heavy pressure.**
9. **Take a few minutes to give the kind of massage the area needs.**
10. **Bring your focus to your open heart, and allow it to pour love and forgiveness into this area of your body. Expand the love to fill yourself entirely with forgiveness and rest in this expanded state of wholeness.**

Journal

Write about your experience.

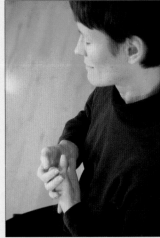

- What area of your body did you choose? Why?
- Jot a quick summary of how and why you distanced from this area.
- What changed so that you want to reconnect with it now?
- How did that area feel when you held it? Did the sensations change as you focused kind attention there?
- What kind of messages did you receive about how it wanted to be massaged?
- What else did you learn?
- How did it communicate?
- To what extent were you able to bring love and forgiveness to this area and to yourself? (Don't expect 100% in one sitting).

This Week

- Spend a few minutes each day with this area, giving it loving touch and listening to its messages about what it wants and needs. Reconnect with it and bring it back into your whole body.
- Notice how this area increasingly becomes incorporated into your awareness of your body as you do different activities, such as walking, sitting, talking, and exercising.

Chapter 12
Supporting Healing
- Choosing Wholeness • Reclaiming Wholeness
- Staying Whole

CHOOSING WHOLENESS

KindTouch provides valuable support when you are ill or injured. This chapter focuses on challenging issues about how to respond when a trauma occurs, or when it remains, and how to be ready if a new illness appears. It is always a choice, whether to split off the problem area or to choose the path of healing which leads to wholeness. When an old injury or illness still feels distanced or unfinished, it is important to reclaim your wholeness. Many of the steps in reclaiming alienated parts of your body have already been explored in previous sections. This chapter will pull it together with the use of the Healing Spiral, massage, and guided imagery experiences to discover your own healing path. The challenge is to find your way to expand your sense of self so that you become large enough to contain all that you are, the difficult along with the fortunate. You can also find the hidden gifts that emerge as you meet your wounded self with acceptance and compassion. KindTouch grounds you in your ability to do this.

Catastrophe awakens us to what we really believe. In the face of illness, injury, or any loss, our choices make the difference between moving toward wholeness and splitting away from some part of ourselves. In the first moments of a trauma this separation feels natural; we don't want to believe we have been hurt. So we distance ourselves from the pain. It then can be easy to fall into a pattern of distancing or denial from that part of our bodies that holds the memory of the trauma.

We can choose to stay whole; to move through the stage of denial, to process all of our feelings about the experience and take care of ourselves. We can realize we are large enough and deep enough to accept a difficult experience without getting lost in it. We can give ourselves the kindness of caring for ourselves while we are ill or injured, and thus maintain our sense of wholeness. If the illness is not severe, we may be able to do this while still taking care of our normal business. But if the trauma is more serious and taking care of ourselves means staying home from work when we feel we must keep going, we must weigh the demands of work against losing our connection to wholeness.

When we get a cold or a small injury, the first inclination for many is to ignore it, wish the problem would just go away, get back to normal, and not be inconvenienced. Sometimes we can get away with this for a while. But if the cold becomes the flu, or the injury hangs on and interferes with our normal activities, we must respond differently.

The most frequent early responses to an illness or injury may be to feel betrayed by our body and to become angry or resentful toward the part that is injured or painful. We distance ourselves from what hurts and think of that part as an "it"—*that* neck is hurting me or *those* painful feet won't let me do what I want. Since it is hurting us, we resent it and don't feel like being kind to it. It's as if an acquaintance had harmed us and, holding onto our anger, we wait for him to make it right. "I didn't do anything wrong. He needs to apologize and fix the situation." This sounds absurd in relation to our bodies, but this is just what many of us do. Ask yourself if you have done this, or are doing it right now. It seems easier to split away from our body than to embrace the illness or injury and pain and realize that we must accept it, take responsibility for it, and care for ourselves.

The cost of splitting off is high. We lose our sense of wholeness. Resisting and fighting a pain or illness means we are fighting ourselves. We don't have to love the illness, but we do need to love ourselves—the-one-who-has-the-illness. We must learn to find a kinder approach so that we may experience our wholeness again. Disconnection within leads to further separations as well—from family, friends, and Spirit, because we are unable to bring our whole selves to those relationships. Thankfully, it is never too late to change; we can choose at any moment to move toward wholeness, whether we are working with a new or an old pain.

None of us escapes illness or injury in our lives. Whether young or old, each of us comes to a time when our bodies no longer do everything we want them to do with the ease and vitality we once had (or wish we had). Physically, we tend to have more issues of discomfort or limitation as we age. Yet, with each experience we have the opportunity to choose our path. We can become more gentle and accepting of ourselves, or we can choose to rail against physical problems and resent our bodies for what they are doing to us. One response leads to more wholeness and peace; the other brings more separation, anger, and fear.

To be whole you must be aware of your choices. When you ignore pain or stiffness in your body, you have made a choice. This option sooner or later probably will bring the consequences of increased pain or a more significant injury or illness. On the other hand, each time you notice a message from your body and respond to it in a kind manner, you will bring yourself closer to healing and expanding your sense of wholeness.

Marc Barasch, in his compelling books, *The Healing Path* and *Remarkable Recovery,* reports that many people who have recovered from an illness against all expectations, or had an unexpected remission, or lived much longer than anticipated, shared certain qualities even though they had very different personalities and temperaments. "...Over and over we took note of a certain quality that we came to call *congruence*—an impression that these people, in the midst of crisis, had discovered a way to be deeply true to themselves, manifesting a set of behaviors growing from the roots of their being." (Barasch, *Remarkable Recovery,* p. 147.) Barasch cites a colleague, Dr. Johannes Schilder of Rotterdam, who also found that seven people who had spontaneous remissions "had emerged from their experience with 'a stronger congruence between emotions, cognition, and behavior.'" (Barasch, p. 147.) I like the fact that they *emerged from their experience* with stronger congruence. This speaks to the growth that illness can stimulate on all levels of who we are. This congruence will manifest in unique ways for each person.

The dominant Western culture does not support this view. First, the idea that healing and health can mean more than just feeling good is foreign to us. Western medicine has a long history of defining health as the absence of disease, where illness and especially death are seen as failures. We have kept doctors in this pattern by handing over our problems to them, then sitting back and waiting for them to fix the problem. Physicians know that many patients are not happy if they leave their office without a prescription. We as a culture are just beginning to change and to

see that each of us is responsible for our own health, that we heal with the *help* of others and through our lifestyle choices.

Another cultural focus that tends to disconnect us from ourselves is our preoccupation with appearance. Many of us value our appearance more than being authentic. This leads to unrealistic expectations of our bodies, both in terms of how we look and how our bodies perform. Our bodies can rarely meet our demands. When they can't, we use self-criticism to motivate change. Authentic growth does not emerge from self-criticism. Expanding your ability to accept and be kind to yourself leads to real growth, with the goal of becoming more deeply true to yourself. Since health is a natural state, your body will tell you what it needs when you listen well.

Our inner voice usually sends gentle messages: "Stop working every hour of the day." "Let's play more." "Choose more pleasurable movement." "Notice when the pain first begins; stretch and relax right away." Your first reaction to such messages may be to see them as frivolous or irrelevant. You may think responding will diminish your outward productivity. It is ironic that these healing messages can be some of the hardest ones to accept.

We can ignore the short term for only so long before the long-term sacrifices begin to occur. At the real bottom line, it is your soul that suffers. It is your soul that you have been learning to know and experience in the exercises in this book. It is from soul that you can bring healing to yourself. Soul is the giver, and your body is the receiver in self-massage. And the body gives the gift right back, allowing you to spend more time in the place of connection and wholeness within yourself, with your place in the world, and with Spirit.

Your choices may lead to improving or curing an illness or injury, but even if not, you can always bring yourself back into wholeness, healing your connection to soul. Each

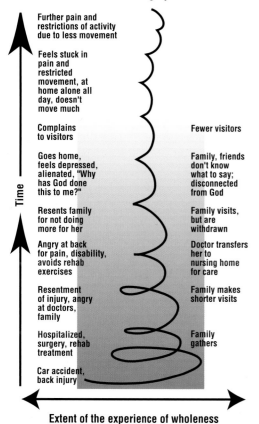

Figure 12-A: Jennifer's Healing Spiral After Back Surgery

Time →

Further pain and restrictions of activity due to less movement

Feels stuck in pain and restricted movement, at home alone all day, doesn't move much

Complains to visitors

Goes home, feels depressed, alienated, "Why has God done this to me?"

Resents family for not doing more for her

Angry at back for pain, disability, avoids rehab exercises

Resentment of injury, angry at doctors, family

Hospitalized, surgery, rehab treatment

Car accident, back injury

Fewer visitors

Family, friends don't know what to say; disconnected from God

Family visits, but are withdrawn

Doctor transfers her to nursing home for care

Family makes shorter visits

Family gathers

Extent of the experience of wholeness

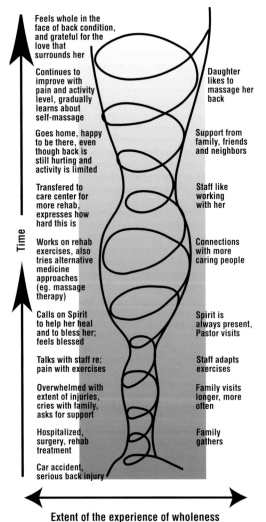

Figure 12-B: Sylvia's Healing Spiral After Back Surgery

Time

Feels whole in the face of back condition, and grateful for the love that surrounds her

Continues to improve with pain and activity level, gradually learns about self-massage

Goes home, happy to be there, even though back is still hurting and activity is limited

Transferred to care center for more rehab, expresses how hard this is

Works on rehab exercises, also tries alternative medicine approaches (eg. massage therapy)

Calls on Spirit to help her heal and to bless her; feels blessed

Talks with staff re: pain with exercises

Overwhelmed with extent of injuries, cries with family, asks for support

Hospitalized, surgery, rehab treatment

Car accident, serious back injury

Daughter likes to massage her back

Support from family, friends and neighbors

Staff like working with her

Connections with more caring people

Spirit is always present, Pastor visits

Staff adapts exercises

Family visits longer, more often

Family gathers

Extent of the experience of wholeness

of us has control over only a certain percent of any problem, and no more. You never know just what that percentage is; it could be as little as 10% or as much as 70% or more. You can make it your intention to heal as much of this problem as possible. Hold the image of your desired outcome, and then let it unfold without judgment. Loving kindness and the intention to heal and to grow are the most helpful things you can give to an injury or illness. This focus will also help you to live well with the condition if it doesn't go away.

The Healing Spiral and Choice

Chapter Three introduced the Healing Spiral and explored its value in discovering the effects different life events or traumas have on us. It gives us a visual way of tracking what happens to our sense of wholeness when we choose to split away a part of ourselves and when we choose the path toward wholeness. Here, we will look at two different responses to the same back injury in two women who took different paths.

Jennifer stayed with her sense of separation after she was injured in a car accident, and constricted to the point that her experience of wholeness became quite limited. See Figure 12A. Her disconnection spread from her resentment about her injuries into other areas of her life, and she became even more isolated. At any point in this constricting cycle she could have made the choice to move toward wholeness, and the spiral would have begun to widen again. In fact, this injury could become the very impetus to find a path toward a greater experience of wholeness.

Many of us find ourselves in a similar position after a tremendous loss. We wake up and see that we have constricted in ways that threaten our well-being in many areas of our lives. Our connections have suffered within ourselves, with family and friends, and with Spirit. The creative moment exists here—at the point when we can choose to reverse the

direction of the spiral from constriction to expansion into greater wholeness. The exercises in this book offer some tools to help you choose and follow the path of greater wholeness.

Sylvia suffered a similar car accident with the same level of injury, but made the choice to move toward wholeness soon after her injuries. With each new challenge she connected with all levels of herself, with her family and friends, and with Spirit to help her find wholeness in the face of chronic pain following her injury. See Figure 12B. Make it your goal to come to a place where you also can respond quickly to even devastating occurrences by bringing all of yourself to a healing path.

Exercise 12a offers an opportunity to create a healing spiral of your responses to an injury or illness. Take the time to consider the choices you have made in the past. The rest of this chapter explores the choice toward wholeness, concentrating initially on how to reclaim your wholeness from an old injury, illness, or pain and then focusing on the challenging path of being ready to move toward wholeness as soon as an injury or illness appears.

HEALING SPIRAL
RESPONSE TO INJURY

Exercise 12a

Introduction

In this journal exercise you have the opportunity to explore one event in your life spiral in more depth.

Preparation

Settle into a comfortable position in the area you've prepared for yourself and begin to turn your focus inward, allowing your eyes to close or to have a soft downward gaze.

Take eight slow, deep breaths, using them to bring yourself fully present. Use the first two to replace tension in your body with softness throughout. With the next two breaths allow your mind to quiet and focus only on being present right now. Let the next two breaths open your heart, feeling the warm light of the love in your heart filling your whole being. With the next two breaths expand your awareness of your soul and your connection with Spirit, sensing the wisdom, love, and healing within and around you.

Let yourself feel grounded as if you had roots that extend down into the nourishing soil. With a sense of peace and comfort, begin the exercise.

DIRECTIONS

1. Choose one time when you were injured, or became ill, or were faced with a great challenge.
2. Note in your journal what the event was, and your feelings at the time.
3. Write the sequence of events after the injury, illness, or challenge.
   a. Did you feel constricted at first?
   b. How long was it before your sense of wholeness began to reappear?
4. Are you aware of moments when you made a decision to move toward wholeness or toward constriction?
   a. How did constricting help you at the moment you chose it?
5. Knowing what you know now, would you change anything?
   a. How has this event contributed to your growth along your healing spiral?
   b. How has your understanding of life and of yourself deepened and expanded?
   c. Has this changed how you see and relate with others?
6. Draw your own healing spiral for this episode.

a. List what occurred during this challenging event on the left side of the page, chronologically beginning at the bottom.
b. Draw your healing spiral, showing how your sense of wholeness constricted and expanded as you dealt with all the consequences from the event.
7. Consider how long the effects of this event lasted and in what ways.
   a. Did the effects catalyze you into growth? In what ways?
8. How has this event contributed to who you are today?

> *There are two ways to live your life. One is as though nothing is a miracle. The other is as though everything is a miracle.*
>
> Albert Einstein

Chapter 12 - *Supporting Healing*

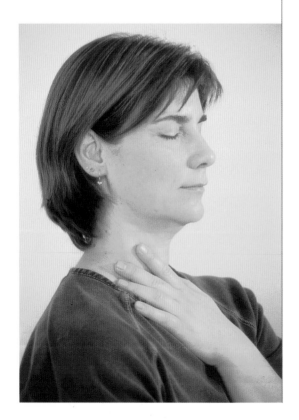

The time to choose wholeness is always now. You may have ignored or rejected an injury or pain or a part of your body in the past, but you can always begin moving back to wholeness at any moment. If you have lost touch with more than one area (or your whole body), working on one part will help the rest at the same time. A lifelong habit of ignoring your body will take time and patience to change, but it becomes easier as you go along. Learning to become softer and more present for one painful part of yourself helps you to be softer and more open toward the rest. As you include more of yourself in your experience of wholeness, it becomes easier to draw in the remaining split-off parts.

Even a temporary restriction in our capabilities creates a significant loss; yet, any restriction can become beneficial to us. An illness or injury can be the very impetus that brings us back to our wholeness. When we are willing to listen to the inner messages from our bodies, we can discover the blessings they bring. They can be messengers telling us about our next step in growth. We do not get an illness or injury *so that* we can grow in a certain direction, but once we are faced with a life-altering condition it becomes part of our path. We can choose to reject it, to fight it, or to accept it; and most likely we will move through a series of such responses. However we work it through, it has the potential for important growth. Such learning rarely comes easily.

Have you ever experienced a friend or acquaintance becoming terminally ill or losing their beloved child or spouse, and because you didn't know what to say you distanced yourself from them and their pain? Few of us can answer "No" to this question. Do you do the same with yourself when you have difficult issues to face? Do you have a bodily restriction or pain that you ignore so that you don't have to slow down or stop? Do you listen when your body speaks in whispers, so

that it won't escalate into even more pain to catch your attention? Bodies tend to make their voices heard; they will speak louder and louder with more pain and increasingly serious conditions until we pay attention. Splitting off from the problem, yearning to get back to life as usual does not help you move forward. Resentment, rejection, and ignoring pain take you further away from comfort, not closer, placing an even thicker layer over the original pain or illness.

When you become aware that you have split off from a part of yourself that has been injured or ill, or that is stiff or painful, what can you do to reclaim it? You can learn to listen and to bring kind touch to yourself, to love and cherish yourself in the same way you do with family or friends who are precious to you. If you stop and spend time with what is hard for you, you can learn to soften your judgments and find the kindness to accept and work with those parts you currently reject. Removing the resistance accesses your ability to care for yourself with grace and love. Going forward involves going through the difficult experience, not around it.

You have already experienced much of the process of reclaiming your wholeness:

1. **Accept the reality** of what you currently reject. Refer to Chapter 10: *Listening to Your Whole Self—Listening, Softening, and Being Present.*
2. **Soften your judgment** about the problem and meet it with kindness. Refer to Chapter 3—*Our Healing Spiral,* and Chapter 11: *Expanding Your Experience of Wholeness—Giving and Receiving, Balancing, and Loving and Forgiving.*
3. **Care for the pain or limitation** with kindness and love. See Chapters 4-9—*Learning the Language of KindTouch* and Chapter 11.
4. **Look for the hidden gift.** See the rest of this chapter including the guided imagery on the *KindTouch CD—Talking with Your Pain,* explained in Exercise 12e.

5. **Expand your connection with Spirit.**
Create a new container within yourself large enough to hold all of your experiences, positive and negative. See Exercise 12c at the end of this chapter and on the *KindTouch CD—Meeting Your Inner Healer.* Chapter 13 explores this aspect further.

You are fine just the way you are.

You don't have to change to be okay; just listen to your whole self and its messages about who you are and what you need. Your path of growth leads to being more true to yourself. Significant physical problems tend to bring up some of our deepest emotional issues—loss of comfort or a cherished role in life, fear of dependence or abandonment, loss of control, and loneliness—to mention a few. These are powerful issues to face and overcome; and yet in spite of all the difficulty, they also bring the opportunity to resolve themselves on a deeper level, leading to more grounded comfort in yourself. Looking at heartfelt issues with generosity helps us to love who we are, instead of always trying to become different or better.

You are fine just the way you are! We all need more self-acceptance, not less. Growth occurs through loving yourself, not through self-criticism. Kindness to ourselves opens a door to greater contentment and a richer life. The exercise at the end of the chapter, *Meeting Your Inner Healer*, also on the KindTouch CD, introduces you to the wise, loving voice of your inner wisdom. Some people say this voice is their higher consciousness, others that it is their soul, or Spirit's voice. You can learn a great deal about what is needed to heal old wounds through this exercise. Your Inner Healer keeps you safe in the process.

Elizabeth Kubler-Ross's stages of coming to terms with dying or other major losses also apply to any significant shift in our physical comfort or capabilities.* The typical first response is shock and denial; we generally think that we should be able to get back to our routines pretty quickly. If this does not happen, we usually get angry or resentful, and wonder why this is happening now, and why to me. It is easy to reject the part of our body that is "doing this to me." With time this all gets pretty depressing, but it is also at this point that much of the work is done to find some peace and acceptance of what is. The struggle helps us learn how to deepen and become large enough to contain this whole new part of ourselves, building on the core of who we are and extending to the outer reaches of our souls. Then we feel whole whether the physical problem is cured or not. This is true healing.

The body can generate a path out of the turmoil of emotions that always accompanies a significant physical problem by giving you the information you need to change your life to become whole. It also returns to you the gifts from KindTouch many times over. When you find yourself stuck in negative or fearful thoughts or emotions, try going to your body. Ground yourself by focusing your heart, mind and soul on blessing your body (see *Self-Blessing* on KindTouch CD) or gently massaging a tender area while giving your whole attention to that area, or simply placing your hands over your heart and breathing in love. When your body becomes calm and you are present in the moment, draw that calmness back into your mind and emotions.

Those who develop chronic illnesses or who have disabilities often are able to come to terms with complex questions about themselves and their lives in this way. When

---

* These are listed as stages, but often only the first stage, shock and denial, occurs predictably in the order presented. Generally people jump back and forth among the stages, depending on their own issues and on what is happening to them.

strength, comfort or independence can no longer be taken for granted, we must reassess who we are and what gives meaning and value to our lives. This process may demand life-changes to become more whole. These changes range from the simple, such as adding a nap in the afternoon, to more complex shifts involving jobs or relationships. Coming to a new understanding of ourselves deepens and enlarges us into feeling whole again (or perhaps for the first time). Thus, working through these difficult steps to come to terms with great losses can result in a gift of immeasurable value.

The Healing Spiral for Reclaiming Wholeness

The healing spiral was introduced in Chapter 3 and was explored more earlier in this chapter. You can now choose to go as deeply as you want into exploring and learning about your own life's healing spiral. Remember that the changing width of the spiral reflects the extent of your *experience* of wholeness. Each revolution of the spiral indicates movement through time and experience. Traumas and losses tend to cause a sudden restriction of your sense of wholeness for a while. It is natural to withdraw and grieve or be angry when trauma or loss occurs. This is part of the healing path. If you acknowledge these needs and embrace your own process, your experience of wholeness will not diminish, even in the worst crises of your life. Trust that your process will heal you. As you grow through the challenges you face, your understanding and realization of wholeness will expand.

The spiral can be helpful in identifying areas of your body you split off and left behind, and which you no longer relate to as integral parts of yourself. Figure 12c demonstrates two possible life events and the resulting constrictions and expansions in one person's sense of wholeness when he lost an important relationship, and later became very

ill. Notice in the second crisis William connected to his wholeness even as his illness progressed.

Do you have unfinished business following a trauma in your background? You can go back to the part of your body that was hurt, and see where you constricted (in your body, and in your mind, heart, and soul). Choose one of the healing exercises in this chapter or earlier chapters to begin to reclaim the wholeness with which you have lost touch.

There are the obvious traumas like major physical injuries or illnesses, loss of loved ones, career disappointments; but less obvious (and more universal) issues can be just as destructive to our sense of wholeness. Consider this list where children and adults can become subject to trauma and loss of self-esteem and disconnection from wholeness.

1. Appearance
   a. Weight: too fat, too thin
   b. Face not fitting the current standard for beauty or good looks
   c. Height: too tall, too short
   d. Too muscular, or not enough
   e. Size of breasts or penis
   f. Hair: too straight, too curly, wrong color
2. Performance
   a. Not chosen for sports team
   b. Loss of identity for athletes who are prevented from playing after an injury.
   c. Low energy or chronic fatigue (invisible inability—"But you look healthy; why can't you do it?")
   d. Uncoordinated or slow moving
3. Any other issues unique to you that you were teased about or felt self-conscious about belong in this list. Identify them and then go back and reclaim yourself again.

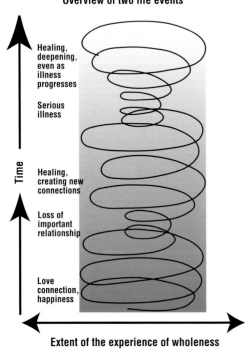

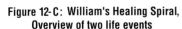

Figure 12-C: William's Healing Spiral, Overview of two life events

Healing, deepening, even as illness progresses

Serious illness

Healing, creating new connections

Loss of important relationship

Love connection, happiness

Time

Extent of the experience of wholeness

HEALING SPIRAL
IDENTIFYING DISCONNECTIONS

Exercise 12b

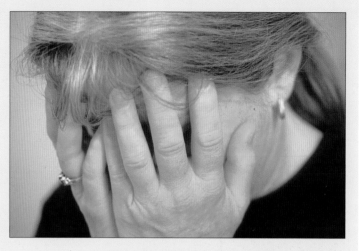

Introduction

The intent of this exercise is to bring you back to yourself with love and kindness, and to gain the perspective that you never stopped growing and moving toward wholeness. Doing this exercise may bring up strong emotions. If it does, find support both from inside yourself and from others—friends, family, spiritual advisor, or a counselor.

If you choose a particularly difficult issue in your life, such as abuse, approach this exercise with great care for yourself. Hold your life in gentle, loving, and wise hands, bringing these gifts to your current self as well as to yourself at the age the problems occurred. Stay clear about how much control you had at the time, and how much you have now. Bring healing to your whole self and reclaim any lost parts of yourself.

It can take a very long time to emerge from devastating events. You may even be in the midst of one right now. It is very difficult to have perspective in the midst of a crisis or large blow to your sense of wholeness. I believe that if your intention is to move toward wholeness, you are doing just that even when you can't see it at the time. It takes hindsight to see how you have overcome great demons. The Hero's Journey always involves a time of feeling lost. If you are in the midst of a difficult time right now, decide whether it is best to do this exercise now to help your process, or later when you have more perspective.

Preparation

Settle into a comfortable position in the area you've prepared for yourself and begin to turn your focus inward, allowing your eyes to close or to have a soft downward gaze.

Take eight slow, deep breaths, using them to bring yourself fully present. Use the first two to replace tension in your body with softness throughout. With the next two breaths allow your mind to quiet and focus only on being present right now. Let the next two breaths open your heart, feeling the warm light of the love in your heart filling your whole being. With the next two breaths expand your awareness of your soul and your connection with Spirit, sensing the wisdom, love, and healing within and around you.

Let yourself feel grounded as if you had roots that extend down into the nourishing soil. With a sense of peace and comfort, begin the exercise.

DIRECTIONS

1. Review your journal notes from Exercise 12a where you identified an injury, illness, or great challenge in your life with which you may have some unfinished business. You can explore this one further or choose another episode that still leaves you separated from a part of your body.
2. If you chose a different issue than you wrote about in Exercise 12a, return to that exercise and answer the questions in your journal about this issue.
3. If you haven't done so, draw your healing spiral for this event.
4. Write in your journal about how you feel separated from the part of your body that was injured, and how this affects your current sense of wholeness. How did your constriction protect you at the time? Is it still needed?
5. Place your hands over that hurt area and hold it in kindness. If you are focusing on emotional pain, notice where in your body you feel it and place your hands there.
6. Listen to what type of touch that area wants and needs now and spend some time giving it. Notice any changes, and adjust your touch to what that area wants. Speak kindly through your hands, and let your body know you want to bring it back into yourself. Invite it to expand and open. Hold it in an imaginary blanket of compassion.
7. Write in your journal about your experience with this exercise. How much were you able to open to this area, and how much did it respond by softening and opening in return?

This Week

- Spend time each day with the part of your body that is affected by the injury you focused on. Give it KindTouch and attention.
- Note your progress in reclaiming that part of yourself in your journal.

GUIDED IMAGERY
MEETING WITH YOUR INNER HEALER

Exercise 12c

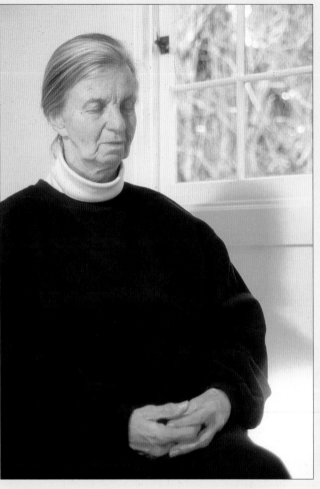

Introduction

This guided imagery will take you through a process in your mind's eye where you can meet and talk with your Inner Healer. You have already learned how to listen to your body's physical messages; now you can add the use of images to hear what your body knows and needs. This is a valuable process because imagery is the language of your soul or higher consciousness, your inner wisdom. When you know how to hear the messages your soul gives you through images, you will have access to great inner wisdom, love, and self-acceptance.

Be aware that sometimes the "inner critic" appears first, posing as a helpful guide. If you hear any messages that aren't kind, loving, and wise, the messenger is probably your inner critic. Thank it for its intention to help, and send it off to rest. Then look further, inviting your Inner Healer to appear.

If you're not sure you can do imagery, just remember the last time you worried about something. Worrying is actually powerful imagery; you use your imagination to paint a vivid picture of what may happen if...(fill in your own topics of worrying). Athletes practice imagery by imagining how they will run the race, or win the game. Planning a party, imagining who will come, what you may talk about, what you'll eat, and so on, all these use strong imagery also.

Tess Taft, in her Complementary Medicine class at the State University of New York at Binghamton, teaches imagery as a powerful means of accessing inner wisdom and love. Her cardinal rules are below:

1. Allow images to come, don't work at it. The greatest mistake is to try too hard; it's like grasping sand—it falls through your fingers.
2. Relinquish all expectations. One mistake is to expect a certain image to form; it's the process of allowing an image to form from beyond your thinking mind.
3. You may see, feel, hear, or sense an image or a response from the image; all are equally good. It's a mistake to believe that if you don't "see" an image you're not doing it right.
4. Be patient; give the image enough time to appear and to respond to you.

Preparation

Gather your journal, pen, the *KindTouch CD*, and your CD player. Have your remote control at hand so you can pause the recording at any point where you want more time. Settle into your comfortable spot and surround yourself with things that evoke safety and sacred space.

DIRECTIONS

1. *Take 3 minutes for a "warm-up" imagery exercise,* using your journal.
   a. Take one minute to write down 5 things that speak to you of healing.
   b. Take half a minute to focus on each image you wrote down. Close your eyes and become aware of what that image says to you about healing.
   c. Write down a brief summary of the message after each image.
2. Think of a question you have about the injury or illness you chose to focus on in the previous exercise, or about a different one.
3. If you choose a challenge in your life, rather than a physical issue, take a minute to notice where in your body you feel the effects of that unfinished challenge.
4. Let your question go and settle into a comfortable position.
5. Relax and listen to the guided imagery, Meeting With Your Inner Healer, on the *KindTouch CD.*
   • If you fall asleep or miss some of the instructions, know that this is just what you need right now. Often your consciousness will absorb the experience like a dream, without your rational brain being aware of the content.
   • If you are awake but the images just don't come to you, relax. This is a skill that develops with practice. You can try this again later, or it may be that other kinds of experiences are better for you. Trust your instincts.

Journal

• After completing the imagery, write about your experience.
• Did you meet with your Inner Healer? Did an inner critic show up?
• Describe your Inner Healer. How did you feel communicating with it?
• What did your healer tell you?
• What messages did your healer have for you about the isolated part of your body (or mind or heart) you have been focusing on? If this issue did not arise this time, plan to meet again with your Inner Healer to learn more about reclaiming your wholeness.
• What did you discover about yourself and your healing path?

This Week and Beyond

• You can meet with your Inner Healer again and again. You can use the CD many times; your experience will be different each time because you'll bring different issues and understandings to the encounter.
• You also can use the first part of the imagery on the CD to move into your special place and contact your Inner Healer, and then turn off the CD, following your own path from there.
• You can meet with your Inner Healer at any time in less formal ways. Simply ask it to appear, and ask a question or begin a dialogue. If this doesn't work, continue working with the CD until you are able to interact with the image on your own.
• Also, you can record this imagery in your own voice using the script in Appendix C.

> *Here, the point of getting well is not necessarily to 'go back to normal,' but to reclaim the soul.*
>
> Marc Barasch

Chapter 12 – *Supporting Healing*

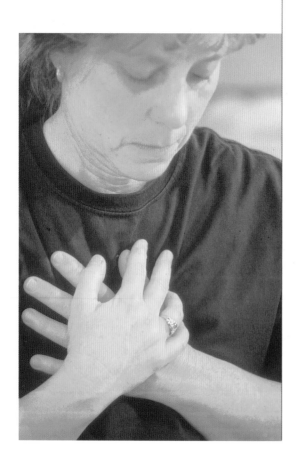

Staying whole with pain and injury, whether short term or chronic, requires special attention. Short-term or minor injuries raise different issues than chronic or severe conditions. Short-term, mild problems bring us face to face with our vulnerability. We live our lives believing we are in control, until suddenly we are hit by something out of our control that interferes with our plans—the flu or a sprain. This reminder of our vulnerability is one of the reasons we tend to get irritated at "minor" illnesses. Chronic or severe conditions also remind us of our vulnerability, but they raise other difficult issues as well. We face significant loss to one degree or another, such as loss of comfort, strength, energy, independence, and possibly some of our roles in life. No longer being able to take these things for granted is itself a great loss and profoundly alters us. The previous discussion, "Reclaiming Wholeness," describes some of the reactions caused by losses related to chronic and severe health conditions.

Staying Whole with Short-term Injury or Illness

Staying whole in the face of a new diagnosis or injury requires that you already have the skills for choosing wholeness and have practiced them enough so that you can bring them into play when you may be feeling overwhelmed and out of touch with yourself. You will need to actively choose the path to wholeness.

When you first become ill or injured, consider whether you are splitting off from the problem. If you are, adequately caring for yourself becomes difficult because you will miss important messages from your illness or the injured area. You cannot listen to your body's messages from a distance. Choose a way to connect to the isolated experience so you can hear what it needs. Then treat it with loving-kindness. Listen to the *Self-Blessing* or do one of the exercises you liked from the

previous sections to help bring yourself back into a sense of wholeness. You may experience resistance to acknowledging the illness or injury, but once you make the shift to acceptance of what is, you will soften within yourself, allowing you to surround the problem with kindness and love. Then you will be able to listen and learn what will help the most. At this point you'll need to answer an important question: Do you want to simply go back to your life as it was, or do you want to use this experience to deepen yourself? If you choose the latter, you can explore some of the issues in the next section on chronic conditions.

Listen to your body! It can tell you what your body needs in order to heal. It may be a transitory episode, which will heal quickly and you can get back to your life. Or it could be that you will need to pay extra attention and give more time to do what is needed to heal. Pay attention to the messages your body gives you. Is this a temporary fluke, or is there a bigger message? Do you need more rest, more quiet time, different foods, more water? Do you need to pay more attention to yourself rather than taking care of everyone else? Do you want to take time for self-massage? Have you been pushing yourself too hard lately or for too long? Do you need some down time? Have you neglected to give yourself good nutrition, good rest, good exercise, good play?

These questions are not raised to suggest you have been doing something wrong and therefore caused your illness or injury. Personally, I find that sometimes the very treatment the illness or injury requires is just what I need for my life in general. If that's the case, I can choose more of that healing behavior in the future without having to get sick to receive it.

Soft Tissue Injuries

Injuries can happen in a couple of ways. First, there is the obvious injury that happens with a fall or a blow. The injury may be apparent at the time of the accident, or it may make itself known over time as the body tries to heal from the trauma. The other type of injury is less obvious but happens more frequently with the repetitive movements required in so

your body and learning how you can move toward healing. Both of these can be used whenever you have questions about these issues.

SOFT TISSUE INJURIES–THE FIRST THREE DAYS

There are other ways of giving yourself KindTouch than by massage. For example, in the first three days of a simple strain or sprain, the traditional wisdom is to follow the "RICE" program: Rest, Ice, Compression, and Elevation. Always consult a medical professional for a diagnosis and treatment plan and follow their advice. These instructions are guidelines for when you've been advised to take this approach.

Rest: The inflammation and the injury process is continuing to form during the first three days (a week or more for serious injuries). Resting the injured area allows healing to begin without further aggravation. Stopping to rest can be frustrating, since often injuries occur just when a person is feeling they must get a lot of things done or when they are in the midst of a strenuous activity they are very invested in. Give yourself the gift of caring for your injury right away so you can heal fully and not carry unnecessary residual impairment.

Ice: Icing helps decrease the swelling and numbs the pain for a while, breaking into the pain cycle, interrupting the escalation of pain. Use a towel between the skin and ice bag and leave for no longer than 20 minutes. Protect the skin from being "burned" by the ice, either from being on too long or by using too little toweling.

Compression: Wrapping an elastic bandage around an area on an arm or leg can help prevent or decrease swelling. It helps an injured joint to stay in alignment, decreasing discomfort. Wrap the bandage so that it is snug without constricting the circulation. If you see swelling below the wrap, it is on too tight.

Elevation: Resting the injured area at a level higher than your heart for an hour once or twice a day and at night helps the circulatory and lymphatic systems to drain the area and minimizes swelling.

You may have noticed that all four of these work best when you use all of them together. It takes resting to elevate a foot, and also to stay still long enough to ice it. The act of wearing a bandage is a good reminder to rest the foot and to decrease its use.

many jobs today. When a muscle group or area of the body is stressed by repetition of the same movements over and over, or is held with tension over a long period of time, there is a slow buildup to a final state of injury that is just as significant as if it had occurred from a trauma. Both kinds of injury need the same approaches to healing.

Two of the guided imagery experiences on the *KindTouch CD* can be very helpful when you're faced with a new problem. *Talking with Your Pain* and *Meeting Your Inner Healer* are powerful tools for hearing the messages from

Staying Whole with Chronic Illness, Pain, or Disability

I have had thirty-two years of chronic pain and I still consider myself blessed beyond measure. I have been thinking about this recently and asking myself how I got here. This book emerged out of the answer to that question.

Chronic pain changes the definition of pain for a person. A person's typical level of pain is gradually redefined as the norm, just as comfort is the norm for others. People with chronic pain often call a sensation pain only if

Marilyn's Story

I've struggled my whole life with the balance between movement from within that's true and movement from without that's imposed. And I do both now. With fibromyalgia the movement I was able to do was so tiny. It was so limited because of my exhaustion and because of my pain that it forced me to become more aware of the subtler movements that I do. I had been doing all these big outward movements to the world and none of the smaller, inner, subtler movements that don't have anything to do with my relationship to the world. They have to do with my relationship to me. When I am moving from my center judgment is gone. There is no judgment, no ego; there's no logical or analytical part of the brain working at all. I don't impose movement. It just comes very spontaneously from somewhere inside. If I'm feeling pain in a certain part of my body, that part of my body may begin moving a certain way. I may lie down on the floor and just begin to feel that pain in that area, and the feeling to do a certain movement arises. It's nurturing. I feel comfortable in myself and in my body after that. It's like after you've had a good cry or a lovely meal or a huge glass of water when you're thirsty. It's that feeling of, "Yes! That felt great."

it exceeds their normal level. Many of my clients with chronic pain say they feel "good" today, simply because their pain is not greater than their constant level. One must listen with a different ear to understand what is meant. Being acutely aware of pain at all times is agonizing, wearying, and depleting for both the individual and his or her family and friends.

When someone has a new, acute pain or illness they respond accordingly; they limit their activities, and often talk about it, receiving sympathy and love from those around them. Typically they gradually recover and return to their usual lifestyle, feeling grateful for healing (or merely take the healing for granted). If the pain or illness and the related behavior go on for a long time, however, it becomes tiresome for them and for those who love them. When pain or illness enters the "chronic" arena, continual focusing on it and agonizing over the difficulties and losses is no longer helpful.

When a condition becomes chronic, make sure causes and diagnoses are accurate, and find treatments (both from external sources and within yourself) that will help. Know what you are dealing with. Both traditional medicine and alternative and complementary approaches can be very helpful. Then it helps to step back and take a realistic look at your strengths as well as the challenges you face.

Gifts from Chronic Conditions

A chronic condition invites (or demands) a reckoning within yourself; you must reevaluate your life and its meaning. It's a time to examine strengths, weaknesses, beliefs, and your sense of value in the world. It's a time when you need to address the value of being rather than doing. In our culture of doing and producing, the ability to be is not generally noticed or admired. But take a minute to think of the person or people you most like to talk to, especially to share things that mean the

most to you. It may be that the reason you trust them and feel comfortable sharing from your heart is because they are able to stop their doing and merely be with you. The ability to hear and be present with other people's painful or difficult experiences or feelings often comes from a person's own experience with pain, illness, or loss. This empathy can be one of the gifts you win from these trials.

Living with chronic conditions is also a powerful teacher about compassion. Being unable to escape from the reality of a painful limitation is a trial by fire that opens our eyes in compassion for all who suffer. It also teaches us that we can survive and even thrive in the face of difficulties we thought we could not live with. This makes it easier for us to be present with others who are also dealing with traumas they are unsure they can face. Chronic illness is an honorable path in life, and offers a difficult but rich road that deepens our souls.

Another gift (a double-edged sword) from chronic illness is that we can no longer take our daily life for granted, or be unconscious of our bodies. Our bodies complain vigorously if we do, and stop us one way or another, sooner or later, from doing what hurts them. This can be frustrating, but also reminds us to care for ourselves kindly.

The exercises at the end of this chapter focus your attention on regaining a sense of wholeness from two different and powerful directions. The first is through bringing your kind touch in a focused manner to a part of your body that is uncomfortable, bringing all you have learned about self-massage (Exercise 12d). The second approach to staying whole in the face of an illness or injury is through guided imagery (Exercise 12e). The use of imagery can be very helpful and powerful with chronic conditions. It allows you to connect with your inner wisdom and loving kindness on an ongoing basis on the path through your altered life. Imagery is the language of the soul, and when messages come from that level of yourself, you know they are true and important. It is a valuable means of learning more about your next steps in healing and staying whole in the face of a difficult life path. Imagery has led me to my most important insights for my healing journey. It can be a surprise to hear what is really needed, and it always feels positive.

Self-Massage

In the middle of a busy life the motivation to massage yourself often comes when pain increases to the point that it intrudes into your daily activities. Then it is tempting to stay engrossed with whatever you are doing while massaging the pain. In this state you will probably go straight to deep pressure on that one area, trying to push out the pain; you will not take the time to listen and gently approach the painful area, understand its cause, and provide healing solutions. We even have a term that encourages us to focus this way; "It hurts good." Unfortunately, this often can be too much direct deep work without a softening introduction to help the whole area calm down first before focusing on one primary spot.

I strongly recommend you try a different approach, one that reminds you that you are whole, one that offers the painful area a way to soften, rather than trying to make it change through deep pressure. The way you begin touching a painful spot affects how the healing processes will be activated within the muscles. Sudden deep pressure causes the muscle to tighten protectively, essentially preventing your fingers access into the muscle. You have to force your way in. On the other hand, if you begin gently with a gliding stroke, the surface tissues begin to soften and relax, letting in your touch. Then expanding to kneading furthers the softening process. When you do more focused massage the muscle now will let you in more easily, and

you do not have to work as hard. Over the years in my massage practice I have come to work more and more gently, and the healing goes as deep or deeper than when I used a lot of pressure. My rule of thumb is to never cause more than mild discomfort. That gives the amount of stimulation to the muscles that is most effective to help them release tension.

Just as in a massage from a massage therapist, the most powerful part of self-massage is the *presence* you bring to your body, to your self. You cannot hear your body's messages or love yourself if your mind or emotions are off somewhere else. You have had practice in becoming present, centered, and grounded as you have moved through the previous exercises. Once you are present you can guide your attention to move into the state you want to bring to your body, one that offers the best of your heart, mind, and soul.

The next step is to *listen;* to feel curious and want to hear the messages held in the painful or stiff area. These messages may be about how that area wants to be touched or held, or they may be about your next step in healing for your whole life. They may be about patterns in your body or in your life that have helped to bring about the tension in that area, or they may be about changes in your life that will help that area to heal. It is curiosity, openness, and an intention to always move toward healing that will help you to hear these messages. The meaning may come as shifts in comfort as you try different kinds of touch, or a new thought may appear that feels true about that area of your life. You may hear words or see an image that gives you important information.

The next step is to help that hurt area to *soften.* This is valuable in itself, but is also vital in helping the area relax enough to let in your more focused touch. Depending on what's going on there this may be a brief step or could be the whole manner in which you touch it. This includes holding, gliding, and kneading.

Nevertheless your best progress can sometimes be made at the darkest time. When there is no humor in sight. When against all logic or sense in body or soul you make the choice to Trust. And learn to say Thank You even on those days.

Margaret McKinstry

> *My body talks to me all the time. But I had to learn to stop and pay attention to it to hear what it says. It's a problem because our minds say so much about our bodies. We're more used to listening to that voice, and the body's talk is so different. It's like the difference between talking to an adult and a child. The adult 'knows,' and the child is exploring.*
>
> Catherine Keir

Finally you bring healing *focus* to the specifics of that area, concentrating on listening with your hands as well as with your mind, heart, and soul. The kind of focusing here is different from an intense, deep pressure trying-to-change-the-problem approach. It is a soft meeting of your self with the painful or restricted area, bringing your open-hearted presence with curiosity and a desire and willingness to move into healing, whatever that means in that moment. It is a presence that allows change, doesn't force it. It is willing to sit with what is, with the pain or the limitation, and holds that experience in gentle hands. It does not leave if the pain does not lighten. In fact, conditions sometimes begin to shift and get better just after the person gives up trying to make things change, and simply finds a way to live a good life with it.

You will have different goals in self-massage depending on the type of illness or injury you have. For short-term problems you will give support to your body while it cures the problem. For chronic conditions your goal is to hold all of yourself in wholeness.

There is much you can do with self-massage for an injury. The way you treat your body helps to strengthen or weaken your healing process. In the first three days, vigorous massage can aggravate the injury; so begin with the simple act of placing your hands over the injured area, giving it kind attention. This can be very powerful. Ask nothing of the injury except to absorb this healing warmth. (See the second step of Exercise 12d: Focusing KindTouch.)

Your body knows how to heal; it is doing just that every minute of your life. Your job is to give it the best environment and support to heal. Your body is always adjusting each system in order to keep you in balance. Food is digested and transported to the cells of the body that need it, such as muscles that are working or healing. Oxygen inhaled by the lungs is distributed to every cell in your body, and carbon dioxide is shuttled back to the lungs and exhaled; other waste products are picked up by the blood or the lymphatic system for removal. If you cut yourself, your body heals the cut. It needs the help of good circulation to bring healing processes to the injured area to prevent infection, bring extra nutrients and oxygen, and take away the extra waste products that form as the body heals. Relaxed muscles in a calm body heal better than tense ones because blood flows much easier when the muscles aren't squeezing tightly around the blood vessels. Good nutrition and drinking lots of water support the body's healing processes. We also can strengthen the healing process a great deal by focusing KindTouch on the injured area.

After several days you can expand the self-massage. Gradually increase into the third and fourth steps of Exercise 12d. Your kind, responsive touch will help you to heal. For illnesses that are short term, listen to what your body wants in terms of self-massage as well as in other areas such as rest and nutrition. Add KindTouch to your other self-care measures.

When you face a life-long (or months-long) difficult condition, you must find ways to minister to your body so that it can do as well as possible, and so that you can maintain your sense of wholeness. Self-massage gives you something you can do to help you stay present and compassionate with yourself. Staying present does not mean you must focus on your pain or restriction all the time. It means finding a way to feel whole, including all of you, the vital and happy parts as well as the painful and restricted parts. Pain speaks so loudly that we tend to forget the other (larger) parts of ourselves that are not in pain. Remind yourself of your wholeness by giving KindTouch to your whole body, creating a container large enough to hold you entirely. Hold the painful area and focus your touch gently. Your goal is not cure, but to give comfort and to bring the painful area into your heart.

Massage Therapy

Professional massage therapists are becoming better recognized for their expertise as health care providers. In Washington State where I work, Washington-based insurance companies are required by law to offer insurance for alternative care. This includes naturopaths, massage therapists, acupuncturists, and nutritionists or dietitians. Insurance coverage is important in order to make massage therapy available to everyone regardless of one's bank balance.

Professional massage therapists know soft tissue (muscles, tendons, ligaments, and other connective tissue) very well and are experts in treating it to aid full recovery. A professional massage therapist uses specific therapeutic techniques to help fully release the muscular effects of an injury so you are not left with residual hypertonicities (overly tight muscles or tendons) that predispose the area to further injuries the next time the muscles are stressed. In chronic conditions professional massage therapists are often the best support you can find. They help your body to stay as soft and flexible as possible, and to keep the restrictions and pain to the lowest level possible. Also, a good therapist will hold you in wholeness, helping you learn how to do this.

Susan's Story

I've always prided myself on being tough and productive and capable, and being a single mom, and having three children and raising them and being a career woman—I had to do everything. I drove myself and forced myself to do things against my body's better judgment, and my body finally said no. I didn't have a choice anymore; I collapsed. Physically I could not do my work and that was devastating to me. Emotionally I had been pushing myself so hard and I felt worthless when I couldn't do it anymore. It really brought me to a horrible time in my life, to face myself and recognize that I couldn't keep coping, as I had been, that I had to change something. I was terrified and threatened by this. I thought I couldn't change anything; I had to do it the way I had been doing it. It turns out I don't have to do it that way. I started changing what I was doing. I didn't do much movement; I couldn't, it hurt too bad. I could barely walk up and down the block without getting exhausted and having to lie down to rest. So I started artwork instead of movement and that really helped. It tuned me in to what was going on inside and softened me a little, to feel the painful things I was feeling and to listen a little more. I had to listen. The exhaustion forced me to listen. And I was moving a little doing the artwork, picking something up, walking from here to there—I was moving a little. Now when I begin moving in the morning, it is more painful to start moving, to begin; but once I get into it and start moving slowly and warming up, I can then do bigger movements without pain. Going slowly, very slowly makes it possible to move without pain. There has to be a kind of continual flowing for me. If I sit too long at my desk without moving, it hurts a great deal to stand, but if I continue moving gently throughout the day, it doesn't hurt more to do bigger movements; in fact it makes it possible. I listen and stay soft and don't let my body freeze up; I involve my body in what I am doing continually.

FOCUSING KINDTOUCH

Exercise 12d

Introduction

In this exercise your hands and fingers will be "melting" into your tissues, moving with gentle curiosity to learn about the muscles. This is a further lesson in tuning into subtleties, and in using your body intuition. You can learn to feel when muscles are tight or relaxed, and when certain spots in a muscle are too tight. Some of these are obvious; most of you will have knots or ropey muscles on the tops of your shoulders and the back of your neck that you can feel. Many areas, though, have subtle signs of tightness. You will use a combination of the sensations within your muscles and the sensations in your fingertips and hands to detect tense spots. The too-tight spots will be anywhere from slightly tender to painful when pressed, giving you feedback about the state of the muscle. If you press hard into these spots, the muscle will brace against the discomfort and won't let in the healing touch. But if you melt your way in, adding pressure only to the point that you detect the first bit of resistance and rest there, you will soon feel the tissue melting slowly under your fingers, inviting your fingers to move in more deeply, but never into pain. Do this with your eyes closed; this amplifies the subtle sensations. Also, gentle rocking of a muscle can help it to soften. Gentle drumming of your fingers or laying your fingers flat over the area and shifting the pressure over the muscle can help also. These are subtle sensations that can take a while to learn. The more you practice the better you'll become. The advantage you have is that you can also shift your attention to how the muscles themselves feel, for additional feedback. This awareness guides your touch.

Preparation

Gather your journal, pen, and oil if you want, or wear comfortable clothes and remove your jewelry. Settle into a comfortable position in the area you've prepared for yourself and begin to turn your focus inward, allowing your eyes to close or to have a soft downward gaze.

Take eight slow, deep breaths, using them to bring yourself fully present. Use the first two to replace tension in your body with softness throughout. With the next two breaths allow your mind to quiet and focus only on being present right now. Let the next two breaths open your heart, feeling the warm light of the love in your heart filling your whole being. With the next two breaths expand your awareness of your soul and your connection with Spirit, sensing the wisdom, love, and healing within and around you.

Let yourself feel grounded as if you had roots that extend down into the nourishing soil. With a sense of peace and comfort, begin the exercise.

DIRECTIONS

1. Select one area of your body that is stiff or painful, that you would like to treat with KindTouch.
   a. Place your attention on being open and curious, very interested in what this area might communicate with you.
   b. Read each instruction and then pause while you do it, noticing the effects in your body.
2. Holding with presence:
   a. Gently place your hand(s) over the area of focus and let them mold to the shape of your body there. If you can't reach the spot, do this in

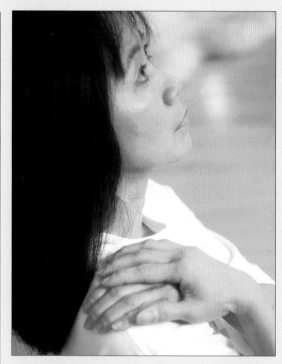

your imagination, and let your muscles experience the sensations as strongly as if your hands were doing the touching.
   b. Accept "what is" (that this area has pain or stiffness right now) and let your hands hold it in loving kindness. Let the warmth of your hands warm the area, and let the pain rest in the love in your heart and soul.
   c. Notice what is happening now that it is receiving your best attention. You may experience shifts in sensation or the area may continue to feel the same. Even if the pain does not change you will be supporting healing in the area and throughout you by creating an experience of your wholeness.

3. Softening, listening
   a. Begin by gently rocking your fingers or hand over the entire painful or stiff area, listening from inside your muscles at the same time you use your fingers and hand to sense any softening in the tissue. This is a subtle practice that may be all that is needed. The longer I practice massage therapy, the more I sense with my fingers, and the less heavy work I need to do. Muscles respond well to a gentle touch that focuses on all aspects of the hurt tissue.
   b. If the muscle wants more touch, begin gliding gently and then more firmly over the whole area. Remember that heavier gliding strokes need to move *toward* the heart.
   c. Add kneading if the area seems ready for it.
4. Focusing:
   a. Let your focus be on your muscles melting into relaxation. Concentrate on your fingers melting gently into the muscle as it lets go. Explore the area from every direction. Give your self some time to be with your muscles in this way.
   b. Ask the area what it needs from you, and simply wait quietly, expecting a response. The answer may relate to how you are touching it now, or about the effect of patterns in your life, or an insight about your next step in healing, or many other messages.
   c. Imagine your hands are having a conversation with the muscles. Let your fingers and hands tell your muscles they are here to listen and to offer healing touch.
   d. Listen for the response in whatever way it comes. The muscle will soften a bit or get that indefinable sensation it gets when it is in the act of relaxing. You may hear words, or see a color, or have a sudden thought that feels true, or feel the rest of your body relaxing, or hear yourself sigh or take a deep breath. Pay attention to your unique response.
   e. When this feels complete, slowly return your attention to the external world with a sense of gratitude for this experience.

Journal

Write about your experience in your journal.

- What did you discover about yourself and the part of your body you focused on?
- What happened when you simply held the area you chose?
- Did you experience any shifts on any level?
- When you asked for messages from your body what kind of responses did you receive?
- Were you able to shift your focus back and forth between doing massage strokes and being receptive to the messages from your body?
- Could you do both simultaneously?
- Did you receive any messages about next steps in healing? About current patterns that may be contributing to your pain or restriction?
- How are your hands and fingers progressing with feeling subtle shifts in the muscles they are touching?
- How do you feel after giving this kind of gentle attention to yourself?

This Week and Beyond

- Spend some time each day this week with the same area of your body you worked with here, developing your sensitivity to hearing its messages. Each time you practice asking questions and then simply listening with the expectation that you'll receive an answer, you will hear better and get an easier flow of information back and forth.
- Focus on other areas of your body when you have a spare minute. Find ways to make this kind of attention a routine part of your day. After you learn how to do it, it doesn't have to take a long time.
- Record your experiences and discoveries in your journal.

GUIDED IMAGERY
TALKING WITH YOUR PAIN

Exercise 12e

Introduction

This guided imagery will take you through a process in your mind's eye where you can meet and talk with a pain or restriction in your body, mind, or heart. You can learn its message and what it needs to bring more wholeness to you. Remember, imagery is the language of your soul, a way to your inner wisdom, love, and self-acceptance. You will be able to come back to this imagery process for any new or changed symptom to know what to do to stay whole.

Preparation

Gather your journal, pen, and the *KindTouch CD* and CD player. Have the remote control handy in case you want to pause the CD to give yourself more time for part of the imagery. Settle into your comfortable spot and surround yourself with things that evoke safety and sacred space. You will be talking to the part of your body that is feeling hurt or isolated.

DIRECTIONS

1. *Take 3 minutes for a "warm-up" imagery exercise,* using your journal.
   a. Take one minute to write down 5 things that speak to you of wholeness.
   b. Take half a minute to focus on each image you wrote down. Close your eyes and become aware of what that image says to you about wholeness.
   c. Write down a brief summary of the message after each image.
2. Play the guided imagery, *Talking with Your Pain,* and relax into the images. The text for this guided imagery exercise may be found in Appendix D.
3. If you get to any uncomfortable spots in this process, invite your Inner

Healer, whom you met in the Exercise 12c, to join you. You can then get the information you need by talking with your healer instead of directly from the pain itself.
4. After completing the imagery, place your hands on the part of your body you focused on. Give it your best KindTouch and thank it for communicating with you.

Journal

Write about your experience in your journal.

- What area in your body did you go to?
- What did it tell you?
- What does it need to become more whole?
- How do you feel after hearing its messages?
- Do you have a plan to follow through on its needs? Why or why not?
- Do you want to meet with this part of yourself through the imagery process again?
- If so, plan a time to do that.

This Week

- Each day spend a few minutes with this area of your body, listening to it and speaking to it through KindTouch and by continuing the conversation you began during the guided imagery.

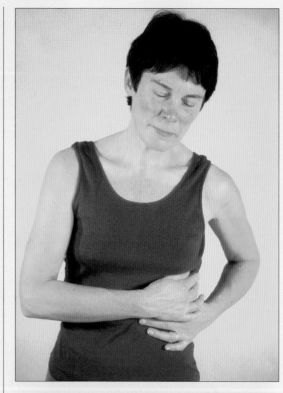

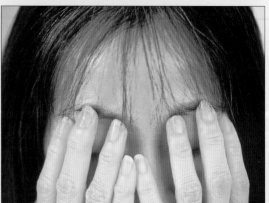

If you enjoy the guided imagery, you can find information to pursue this interest in the Resource Section at the back of the book. As well as books and tapes, you can locate interactive imagery practitioners who can work with you individually to access your inner wisdom for your life.

Chapter 13

Embodying Spirit

- Expanding Your Experience of Spirit
- Grounding Spirit

EXPANDING YOUR EXPERIENCE OF SPIRIT

Our connection to our spirituality is often abstract, something that we retreat from our active life to experience. I am interested in how we can bring our sense of Spirit and connectedness into our active lives. A mountaintop experience of Spirit is great, but so often when the retreat or the church service is over we go back to another (busier) part of ourselves that is not firmly connected to the divine. This is where we spend most of our time, rushing to get everything done, to spend time with the kids, to go to work and do the housework and pay the bills, and so on and so on; and at the end of the day we feel like we ran a race in which the finish line was constantly being moved farther away.

Our life is a mystery and a miracle. It's beyond our ability to fully comprehend it, but if we open ourselves to it we can have a direct experience of it. You've already experienced yourself in wholeness through bringing KindTouch to your body. It takes only a slight shift of attention from there to sense how you belong in the world and to feel as if you're resting in the hand of Spirit. This kindness emanates first from that which created us, Spirit. We simply do our best to come into Its presence.

One of the most important questions in life is how to stay conscious of our souls while we are living our busy lives. Grounding our spirituality in our bodies is a great route to doing this. By massaging our own bodies we bring our hearts and souls to ourselves in a very concrete way, and soon find that this quality of being kind to ourselves spills over into other parts of ourselves too.

When my body experiences and receives my kind touch, I carry that kindness with me, firmly grounded in my body. When my inner critic voices its judgments it lands on less fertile soil. There is a physical part of me that knows and likes my kindness and objects to the judgment, bringing this previously automatic process of self-criticism to awareness. It also offers an alternative; I often find myself stroking my chest over my heart when I'm feeling stressed about something I've done or not done, and I allow myself to receive that gentle acceptance and kindness. Then this bodily experience of kindness can expand to help quiet my mind and soften my heart. Then of course I'm in a better position to be present for others also, since I'm not in a defensive mode of being.

If we can find ways to experience the miracle of our lives firsthand, we can be filled with awe and gratitude. The more I have learned about the human body in my studies and work as a nurse and a massage therapist, the more I wonder how it is that almost all babies are born with everything working perfectly. Even as we age so little goes wrong compared to the vast complexity of what we are. Learning about even one system in the body, or looking at how even one cell works fills me with awe. All the cells, organs, and organ systems work in total harmony with each other. The intricacy and complexity of the creation that is humankind is way beyond my comprehension. Beyond that, the myriad other species of animals and plants, the structure of the earth, the air and atmosphere, and how they all move together so seamlessly as a whole expands my awe even more.

It's the ability to be present in a moment that allows us to consider these things. We need to learn to be present in each moment; that will increase our connection to what we value and to Spirit. The miracle that is life can be experienced directly, through a heartfelt and soul-filled connection with our bodies, with all that is around us, and with Spirit. As we spend more time perceiving abstract ideas and feelings in the grounded way that our bodies offer us, the experience will grow in the other direction too–up from our bodies into our hearts and minds. Our souls already know all this; they are merely waiting for us to notice and make room for them. Then Spirit will truly be a part of us, and we will carry this connection with us everywhere. When we experience and know ourselves on every level we also gain a sense of our unique place in the world.

Perhaps everything that frightens us is, in its deeper essence, something helpless that wants our love.

Rainer Maria Rilke

FINDING SPIRIT IN YOUR BODY

Exercise 13a

Introduction

Massaging your own body while listening to your body's sensations and wishes has brought you into contact with all of yourself–body, mind, heart, and soul. You have experienced yourself as giver and receiver at the same time. You have listened, softened, loved, and forgiven in the exercises in this book. You have explored your healing spiral and expanded your experience of wholeness. The power of presence grows with practice and allows us to be aware of all these aspects of ourselves at the same time. It takes only a slight shift of attention to feel ourselves resting in the hand of Spirit.

Preparation

Settle into a comfortable position in the area you've prepared for yourself and begin to turn your focus inward, allowing your eyes to close or to have a soft downward gaze.

Take eight slow, deep breaths, using them to bring yourself fully present. Use the first two to replace tension in your body with softness throughout. With the next two breaths allow your mind to quiet and focus only on being present right now. Let the next two breaths open your heart, feeling the warm light of the love in your heart filling your whole being. With the next two breaths expand your awareness of your soul and your connection with Spirit, sensing the wisdom, love, and healing within and around you.

Let yourself feel grounded as if you had roots that extend down into the nourishing soil. With a sense of peace and comfort, begin the exercise.

DIRECTIONS

Focus on one hand, and notice all you can about how it is structured.

1. Notice how the bones and joints fit together and how the muscles and tendons are attached so that you can move easily.
2. Move your hand and fingers and become aware of how these systems work seamlessly together for a smoothly functioning hand.
3. Become aware of how each cell is nourished from the blood that flows along the rivers of your circulatory system, keeping all the bones, joints, muscles, and skin healthy.
4. Recognize that there is a rich network of nerves that allows your fingers to have detailed sensitivity, and that lets you move your hand and fingers in the ways your mind directs.
5. Massage your hand for a minute, soaking in the rich variety of sensations you are capable of experiencing.
6. Spend a minute thinking of all the things your hands do for you.
7. Now open your heart to your hand, letting your loving kindness encircle your hand, giving gratitude for all it is and does for you.
8. Notice how that opening affects your hand's sensations and how it affects your mood and feelings.
9. If your hand has any discomforts or restrictions, hold these in kind acceptance as part of the whole.
10. Ask your soul to be present, and become aware of it inside and also surrounding your hand and your body, and notice what happens.
11. Focus on the interrelation of all things and beings. Your soul gives you a large enough container to hold this expanded awareness.
12. Let yourself be aware of the miracle

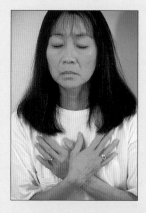

that you are and the mystery that is life.
13. Ask yourself what your unique place or gift in the world is, and allow an answer to appear.
14. Allow your awareness to expand to be in touch with Spirit, always present and waiting for us to open to It.
15. Spend a minute enjoying all you've been experiencing.
16. Bring your attention back to the room, stretching and inviting a sense of invigoration to fill your body.

Journal

Write about your experience in your journal.

- About your body.
- About yourself as whole.
- About your relationship to all life.
- About your unique gift or place in the world.

This Week

- Spend a few minutes each day focusing on one part of your body, bringing in your awareness of the many systems that bring it life: bones, muscles, circulation, and nerves, and so on. Let yourself rest into a deeper sense of your connection with all of life, and of your unique gifts and place of belonging in the world.

Chapter 13 – *Embodying Spirit*

I invite you to think about how you will incorporate KindTouch and a deep experience of yourself as whole into your busy life. It takes conscious intention to create a healing path. By reviewing your journal notes to identify activities that are most meaningful to you, you then can create your own practice to deepen your healing journey. Build on the exercises in this book or create your own practice. Just continue to treat yourself kindly. I believe this is a lifelong practice of noticing what is happening inside yourself and then bringing kindness from your body, heart, mind, and soul to each part of yourself, just as you would for your most cherished companion. All you need is your conscious intention to always be moving toward healing and a desire to bring KindTouch to yourself.

KindTouch can become a healing practice that will bring you to a grounded experience of vital inner gifts:

- The ability to be fully present
- Feeling a deep and loving connection with your true self
- Knowing yourself as whole
- Experiencing your whole self as a unique one-of-a-kind miracle
- Feeling the grace of giving-and-receiving within yourself
- Knowing how you belong in the world
- Experiencing a deep connection with Spirit.

We only need to bring a listening presence consistently to our bodies and we will receive from them a path toward these gifts.

The lists below summarize the key themes in this book. Exercise 13b at the end of this chapter offers suggestions for creating a lifelong self-massage practice.

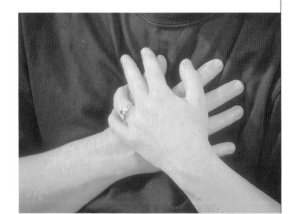

Guidelines for KindTouch:

1. Come present—body, mind, heart, and soul.
2. Bring the best of your heart, mind and soul into your hands to minister to your body.
3. Work with attentive awareness as both giver and receiver.
4. Keep a listening focus in your muscles and whole body.
5. Trust your own body wisdom to guide your self-touch, focusing on subtle body sensations.
6. Work gently and invite the body to soften and relax, rather than trying to force change.
7. Move from a broad, gentle focus to a more specific and focused touch for painful spots, melting into the muscle as it softens.

Principles of a healing path

1. Life is seen as a healing journey with every experience contributing to growth and deepening, rather than judging experiences as good or bad and rejecting all the bad or difficult parts of life.
2. For all us who live in a body, there is a natural flow back and forth between comfort and pain, ease and challenge.
3. Healing and growth can emerge out of a difficult time.
4. Health is seen as wholeness, rather than part of the cure/failure model.
5. Healing means following the path toward an expanded experience of wholeness.
6. Wholeness includes body, mind, heart, and soul.
7. The myth that wholeness is only happiness is replaced by reclaiming all of yourself—pain as well as pleasure.
8. The healing spiral can be used to look at a day, at a challenge, at an illness or injury, or at your whole life. The spiral widens as your experience of wholeness expands, and narrows when you constrict and forget that you are always whole.

9. The power of congruence among body, mind, heart, and soul leads always to wholeness, and sometimes to cure.
10. For any illness, injury, or challenge a person has an unknown percentage of control. Approach each by holding your desired outcome as your intent, and then let it unfold without judgment or attachment to outcome.
11. The real bottom line is not money and status; it is soul and connection with Spirit.

Keys to reclaiming wholeness

1. There is a choice to be made at each point in an illness, injury, or challenge—between the path toward wholeness and that of separating the painful part from yourself. This choice can be made at any moment, even long after the injury.
2. Illness or injury can be the very impetus that brings you back to yourself.
3. Listening to the messages in symptoms gives an understanding about the effects of your life patterns and what is needed for healing.
4. The point is not to "try to change" your self to be "better," but to embrace more of yourself as you are.
5. The path of reclaiming your wholeness requires that you:
   a. Soften your judgment about the problem and meet it with kindness.
   b. Accept "what is" that you currently reject.
   c. Care for the pain or limitation with kindness and love.
   d. Look for the hidden gift— see symptoms as messengers about next steps for growth and healing.
   e. Create a new container or context for yourself and the illness—a larger one that holds all of your experiences in kindness.

Keys to staying whole in the face of a new injury, illness, or loss

1. Healing involves choosing the path of moving toward wholeness, flowing through all of the experience, not rejecting parts of yourself.
2. KindTouch gives you something to do to move toward healing and wholeness, even in the early, numb phase of response to a large loss.
3. The path involves listening to your body and its needs, and responding with kindness.

Gifts from chronic conditions:

1. Any illness, but especially chronic conditions, offers an opportunity to deepen your being, expanding the soul of who you are.
2. Even though uninvited, chronic illness is an honorable life path, one that deepens heart and soul.
3. Illness urges you to reevaluate your life and what brings you meaning and happiness—to look at the balance between being and doing.
4. A profound gift from chronic health problems can be the development of empathy and compassion for yourself and others, the ability to be with those who are suffering.
5. You can no longer take your daily life patterns for granted, but must become aware. This gift is a reminder to treat yourself kindly.

We see that when the activities of life are infused with reverence they come alive with meaning and purpose.

Gary Zukav

CREATING AN ONGOING
SELF-MASSAGE PRACTICE

Exercise 13b

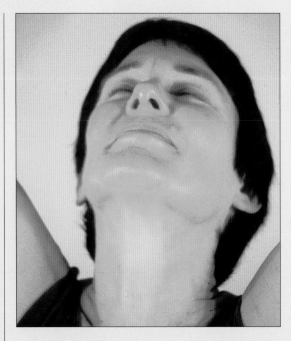

Introduction

Create your own practice based on your experiences with the exercises and themes of this book. Deepen your experience by reviewing your journal notes for the exercises, and find the ones that gave you the most vital experiences—the ones you want to do again. Perhaps you will choose the exercises that stimulated new ideas of ways to move along your healing path. Or you may identify experiences from your life that you want to explore further. Use the following list of ideas to create a lifelong self-massage practice.

DIRECTIONS

1. Find some way to bless yourself every day. Use the *Self-Blessing* on the *KindTouch CD* or develop your own.
2. Use movement to remind you of the life in you and of how your body likes to move.
3. Find ways to give yourself massages, short or long, for areas that hurt and for ones that feel terrific. Use the *Guided Self-Massage* on the *KindTouch CD* as often as you like.
4. Make listening to your body a habit. Listen while you massage and when you are moving.
5. Find ways to soften your body, your judgments, your heart, and to give loving messages (and massages) to yourself and your body.
6. Become deep enough and large enough to be able to hold all of yourself, pleasure and pain—to experience your wholeness throughout the day.
7. Incorporate your awareness of both giving and receiving into all your activities.

8. Add the awareness of gratitude to each day—for your body and for your life.
9. Give yourself the gift of play and creativity in some way that adds energy to your life.
10. Think ahead about how to respond to things that throw you off balance, how to flow through them in ways that support your wholeness.
11. Plan ahead based on what you learned about what you need when you are hurt, so you can hit the ground running in terms of being kind to yourself if you get sick or injured.
12. Focus your attention and KindTouch on painful areas.
13. Continue to think of your life as a healing journey, not judging but opening to every kind of experience each day.
14. Consider how you will bring Spirit into your daily, physical life.
15. Use imagery to tap into your inner wisdom and love. Use the *KindTouch CD* imageries, *Meeting with Your Inner Healer* and *Talking with Your Pain*, or do it in your own way.

This Week and Beyond

- Keep your written plan with you until it becomes an automatic part of your life.
- Revise it as you find what works well and what doesn't fit after all.
- Review your plan periodically and take the time to listen to your inner wisdom for your next steps.
- Plan to spend time reviewing your plan every month or every quarter, to update how each area of your body likes to be touched, to note your progress in your healing journey through life, to deepen

your experience of yourself as whole, and to remember what is most important to you.

- At the end of one year and the beginning of the next, rather than making isolated resolutions, take stock of where you are on your healing journey and discover what your next step in growth is. Make that your spiritual intent for the year.

I belong to a women's sacred circle where every year we each state our spiritual intent for the year. You won't be surprised to hear that for the past year mine has been "I soften." I have used this as an affirmation every morning, a balm when I am tense, and a path to the center of my true self. I invite you to identify a spiritual intent for yourself, and allow it to work its magic in your life.

Blessings on your journey!

Appendix

Settle into a comfortable position and begin to turn your focus inward, allowing your eyes to gently close. Take a few deep breaths and let them be letting-go breaths. Let yourself float on your breath, feeling your body rise a bit when you inhale, and settle with your exhalations. Each time you do this blessing you can sink deeper into your experience.

I'll lead you through eight slow, deep breaths, focusing on two at a time. You can use these to bring yourself fully present. With the first two breaths focus on releasing your body; inhale softness and exhale physical tension. Let your body sink deeply into the support you're resting on. The next two breaths are for quieting your thoughts. Let your mind become quiet. Release any extraneous thoughts, and bring your focus inward. Let the next two breaths open your heart; see or feel the warm light of your heart's love spill over and fill your whole body with warmth and compassion. Release any other emotions. With the next two breaths expand your awareness to your soul and your connection with Spirit, opening to the tenderness, support, and healing within and around you. Allow your breathing to become easy and relaxed while you rest in the stillness and acceptance that encompasses your body, mind, heart, and soul. Again, let your body float on your breath, feeling it rise a bit on the in-breath, and settle with your out-breath. Let yourself feel grounded as if you have roots that extend down into the nourishing soil.

Now place your hands over your heart and feel them fill with the light from inside you. Know that you are blessing yourself now, bestowing kindness, healing, and light. Bring your hands to your face, for a moment resting them over your face in a blessing. Gently stroke your fingers several times from the center of your face outward, feeling that kind touch on your skin. Placing your hands on the top of your head, stroke down to your shoul-ders several times, moving across the back and sides of your head and neck. Let yourself receive the healing and love your hands are bringing to yourself.

Place each hand on the opposite shoulder and stroke down your arms to your hands several times, letting your hands conform to the shape of your arms and turning your palms to face each other. Let your arms and hands focus on receiving your kindness and gentle touch.

Stroke your hands down the front of your body several times, over your chest, your abdomen, thighs, legs, and feet. If you don't want to reach that far, send your touch through your imagination. Notice the effect of bringing loving touch and healing energy in a flow through your body. Just notice how your body feels as you bring these qualities to yourself.

Now let your hands relax in your lap, and let the blessing flow throughout your body, including all your organs. And now feel that kind touch and healing energy flowing down your back, across your shoulder blades, down your ribs to your low back and buttocks, and down the sides and backs of your legs to your feet. Rest your attention over your feet for a moment; thank them for all they do for you, and bless them.

Now rest your hands in your lap and bless your whole body with gratitude, for all it is and does for you, and all it's been through with you. Notice how your body feels. If any area is uncomfortable or stiff, place your hands over that area, or imagine your hands there, and offer acceptance, love, and healing energy. Bring your full presence to surround this place. Allow the area to receive this soft-ening and to float on your compassion and healing support.

Now bring your attention to your wholeness—your body, mind, heart, and soul as one. Let each part of yourself soak in the healing and the love that is surrounding you right now. Let yourself rest in the blessing you have been giving yourself, and in your healing connec-tion with Spirit.

And now begin to come back to the external world around you. Be aware of the support of the surface you're resting on, and notice any sounds around you. Allow an enlivening energy and spirit to fill your body and to fill your heart, your mind, and your soul, so that you can move into your day, or rest into your night, bringing this blessing with you. If you'll be getting up and moving, open your eyes when you're ready, and stretch your whole body like a cat to mobilize your energy for your day. If you'll be sleeping, let your whole body sink in to the rest and support offered by the surface you're lying on, and sleep well.

Appendix B: Whole Body Relaxation Massage–Exercise 9
Script for Guided Self-Massage #2–KindTouch CD

Settle into a comfortable position, and take a few deep breaths and let them be letting-go breaths. Let your body float on your breath, feeling it rise a bit on your in-breath, and settle more and more on each out-breath. Bring your attention inward, becoming aware that you'll not only be massaging your body, but also greeting yourself, and both giving and receiving kind touch. Let your intention be to bring the best of yourself to this massage, and to openly receive its gifts.

Take a deep breath, and begin by gliding your fingers over your forehead several times, ending with circles over your temples. Then continue gliding over your cheeks and jaw, ending with circles over your jaw muscles. Then use the tips of a couple of fingers to move back and forth under your cheekbones, greeting those muscles that can be tight, bringing them some gentle circles, moving down the muscles to your jaw bone, encouraging them to soften and let go. Glide over your throat. Now "shampoo" your scalp, making circles or back and forth motions, letting yourself feel how nice it is to experience this kind of touch. Now grasp your earlobes, squeezing while you move your thumbs and fingers in opposite directions, working your way around your ears. Complete the massage for your face and head by using the surface of your palms and fingers to glide over your whole face, over your scalp, and down over your neck. Then do nerve strokes over your face and throat by gently drawing your fingertips across your skin, noticing how relaxing that is, not only for this area but also for your whole body. Take a slow, deep breath and soak this in.

Now move to your neck and shoulders. If you're using oil, apply it now to your neck and both shoulders...Use this time to bring your kind attention to this area. Beginning at the top of your neck with both hands, glide down the sides of your neck across your shoulders, and then down the back of your neck and shoulders, noticing how these muscles feel today. Then walk your fingers down the center of the back of your neck, making circles or back-and-forth motions as you move along close to the bones. Repeat these walking strokes twice more, moving farther to the sides each time. Now move to the muscles on the top of your shoulders. Place one hand on top of the opposite shoulder, and relax the shoulder you'll be working on. Knead that area by pulling your fingers up toward the heel of your hand. Then walk your fingers across the top of your shoulder, making circles or back-and-forth motions with them. Then move to the other shoulder and repeat the kneading for that muscle, making sure you let this shoulder and arm relax. Now walk your fingers across the top of your shoulder, making small circles or back-and-forth movements over them. Use your imagination to spread this sensation from both shoulders down into your back. Then place the fingertips of both hands just below the base of your skull, and beginning toward the middle, move your fingers back and forth over the many muscle attachments here, moving out to the sides, rocking back and forth over each spot before moving on. Work up onto the surface of your skull a bit also. Complete the work in this area by gliding down again over the sides and back of your neck and shoulders; and then do gentle nerve strokes with your fingertips in the same path, letting your fingers float off the edges of your shoulders, and inviting the softening to go even deeper. Take a moment to notice your sensations.

Now move to one arm and start by applying oil if you're using it. Direct your breath and your kind attention to your arm. Rest your receiving arm in your lap so it can fully relax. Begin at the outside of your wrist, and glide firmly up to your shoulder, gently gliding back down. Then glide up the inside surface of your arm, preparing the muscles for more focused touch. Glide back up to the front of the muscle that wraps around the top of your arm, and knead it all the way around to the back, lifting your fingers toward the heel of your hand. When you reach the back, move down, kneading the muscle in the back of your upper arm, and then glide back up. Then rest the arm being massaged along your thigh, palm up; and starting at the shoulder, knead the muscle in the front of your arm, moving down to your elbow, and gliding back up. Now move to the top of your forearm, kneading the outside from elbow to wrist, lifting your fingers toward the heel of your hand and remembering to let your receiving arm stay relaxed and limp, glide back up. Now knead the inside of your forearm, and glide back up. Take a moment to notice how your arm feels, receiving this kind touch.

Now, starting at your elbow, use the pads of your fingers to rock over the muscles on the outside of your forearm, moving down to your wrist, and then gliding back up. Now do the same for the inside of your forearm, using your fingers or thumb to rock across your muscles. Notice how your muscles feel with this more focused stroke, and adjust your pressure accordingly.

Now move to the palm of your hand, and use your thumb to do a series of focused glide strokes, moving from the heel of your hand to the base of each finger and thumb. Then grasp the muscle in the web between your thumb and hand, and roll back and forth across this muscle. Now squeeze and rub each finger between your thumb and fingers, covering all sides; move from one finger to the next, including your thumb. Let each finger relax, and notice how your whole hand begins to feel warmer and softer, and filled with energy.

Finish this arm and hand by gliding up all the surfaces of your arm, noticing how your arm feels, receiving this massage. Then do gentle nerve strokes down each side of your arm, gently drawing your fingertips from your shoulder to your hands, and moving off the ends of your fingers. Invite the calming effect of this to spread to the rest of yourself, too. Notice how this arm feels. Does it feel different from your other one? Enjoy the gifts you have given yourself.

———————————

Now use this hand and arm to give the same gifts to your other side. Begin by spreading oil if you're using it; and let the receiving arm rest in your lap while you turn your attention to it. Glide up each side of your arm with a firm touch, returning to your wrist with a lighter gliding stroke each time. Move to the muscle that circles the top of your arm, and starting at the front, knead your way around to the back, lifting your fingers toward the heel of your hand. When you reach the back, continue kneading down the muscle in the back of your arm to your elbow, and glide back up. Knead the muscle on the front of your arm from shoulder to elbow, and glide back up. Now move to your forearm at your elbow, kneading the back first, working down to your wrist, and gliding back up; and then knead the inside of your forearm, and glide back up. Coming back to the outside of your forearm at your elbow, rock back and forth over the muscles, using the pads of your fingers or your thumb, moving down to your wrist, glide back up to your elbow; and repeat this rocking stroke over the inside of your forearm, using your fingers or thumb, and gliding back to your elbow. Now move to your hand. Glide your thumb across the palm of your hand from the heel to each finger and thumb using the amount of pressure your hand likes the best. Squeeze the muscle in the web between your thumb and hand, and roll back and forth across this muscle. Now squeeze and rub each finger between your thumb and fingers, covering all sides. Notice how your fingers feel, receiving this attention.

Let your fingers and hand soak this in. Finish by gliding up all sides of your arm; and then doing light nerve strokes down your arm and hand, and off the ends of your fingers. Take a slow breath and soak in the pleasure.

———————————

Moving to your torso, begin by applying oil if you're using it, over your chest and abdomen, and as far as you comfortably can reach over your sides, low back, and hips. Use your hands to glide down over the center of your chest and abdomen to your hips. Repeat this twice more, moving to the sides of your ribs. Then place the heel of one hand on the center of your chest, and glide upward and outward toward your shoulder several times. Grasp this large chest muscle at the front of your armpit between your fingers and the palm of your hand. Knead it by pulling your fingers up toward the heel of your hand or the side of your thumb, moving along the muscle toward the center of your chest, avoiding breast tissue. Now continue kneading around the side of your ribs, kneading the muscles as far onto your back as you can comfortably reach, and moving down to your waist. Use your imagination to spread this sensation across your back. Now glide the heel of your other hand from the center of your chest up to the opposite shoulder. Grasp your chest muscle and knead it, moving from the front of your armpit toward the center of your chest and gliding back out; and then knead your way around onto your side and back, moving down to your waist and gliding back up. Now glide in a circle around your abdomen, making sure that you come up the right side, go across under your ribs, and then down the left side, so that you go with your bowel, not against it. Now bring your hands around to your low back as far as you comfortably can reach, and glide down and across your buttocks. Bring your hands back up to your low back, with the palm of your hands against the skin.

Knead each side alternately, squeezing one hand and then the other as you move down across your back and buttocks to the sides of your hips, lifting your fingers toward the heel of your hand. Then glide from your low back across your buttocks. Now reach around again to your sacrum (just below your spine), and pressing the tips of your fingers inward, move them in circles as you progress up the sides of your spine, only as far as you comfortably reach. Finish by gliding once again over your low back and buttocks, and then over your chest and abdomen, and down your sides and hips.   Follow this with nerve strokes, gently stroking down and off the sides of your hips. Take a slow deep breath and soak in the relaxation.

———————————

Now, moving to your legs and feet: Place one foot on a stool, or get in a comfortable position to work on your leg. Apply oil to one leg and foot, and focus your kind attention on it. Then starting with your hands on the top and bottom of your foot, glide up onto your leg to your knee. At your knee, place one hand over the other to give firmer pressure for the large thigh muscles, and glide up the outside of your thigh; when you reach your hip, glide gently back to your knee and glide up the front with a firm touch, and down with a lighter one, then the inside, and then the back. Then, starting at the hip on the outside of your thigh, use both hands to knead from your hip to your knee, and glide firmly back up; knead the front of your thigh from hip to knee and glide back up with a firm touch; knead the inside of your thigh; and glide back up, and then when you reach the back, knead all the way down your leg to your ankle. Then glide back up your whole leg. Moving to the outside of your leg at your hip, explore the muscles right around the hipbone by moving your fingertips back and forth in a circle around that bone; and then expand your movements to explore your whole hip and buttock area with this cross-fiber friction—just get to know what those muscles feel like, all the way up and around to the bones where they attach; work on tender areas more gently and with flatter fingers. These muscles don't get massaged often; just notice how they feel when they receive KindTouch. Now moving to just below your knee, to the outside of your shin bone, make alternating circles with the fingertips of both hands, moving down from knee to ankle. Do a firm glide back up that muscle. Moving to your ankle, make alternating circles with both thumbs around your ankle, and over the whole sole of your foot, moving out to your toes and squeezing each toe.

Then run your thumb from your heel to the base of each toe in 5 strips, to cover the whole surface. Complete this leg by gliding back up all sides, and then lightly doing nerve strokes down to your foot and off the tips of your toes. Take a breath and notice how this leg feels compared to the other one.

Moving to your other leg, spread the oil first, if you're using it and direct your attention to your leg; then place one hand on each side of your foot and glide up to your knee; and then use one hand over the other to firmly glide up the outside of your thigh, returning to your knee with a gentle glide. Glide up each side of your thigh, remembering to use firm pressure going up your leg and gentle pressure going back down.

Then starting at your hip on the outside of your thigh, use both hands to knead your way down to your knee, and then glide back up. Knead down the front of your thigh and glide back up. Repeat this for the inside surface of your thigh, and notice how your leg feels receiving this kind touch. When you reach the back, continue kneading all the way down to your ankle; and glide all the way back up. Move to your hipbone at the outside of the top of your leg, and use your fingertips to move back and forth over the muscles attached in a circle around this bone. Then expand your circles to explore your whole hip and buttock, upward and backward to the bones these

muscles attach to. If you find tenderness, lighten your pressure, or change from your fingertips to the flats of your fingers, and gently offer a softening touch.

Now, moving to just below your knee and just to the outside of your shin bone, make alternating circles with the fingers of both hands as you move down to your ankle, gliding back up in a firm glide. Now make circles with your thumbs around your ankle and over the whole sole of your foot, moving out to your toes, and squeezing each toe. Then run your thumb along the sole of your foot from the heel to the base of each toe, covering the whole surface. Glide up all sides of your leg, and then finish with light nerve strokes down your leg to your foot and off your toes. Take a breath and relax your whole body.

Complete your whole massage by doing nerve strokes from head to toe, to remind you of your wholeness and to calm your whole system. And now let yourself notice the relaxed but vibrant energy you can feel from massage.

Let this energy grow into comfortable warmth. And slowly move back into your day, and enjoy.

Appendix C: Meeting with Your Inner Healer–Exercise 12c
Script for Guided Self-Massage #3–KindTouch CD

Settle into a comfortable position and begin to turn your focus inward, allowing your eyes to gently close. Take a few deep breaths and let them be letting-go breaths. Let yourself float on your breath, feeling your body rise a bit when you inhale, and settle with your exhalations. Take a moment to be aware of a question or concern about your health for which you'd like to receive some kind wisdom. Then let that issue go.

I'll lead you through eight slow, deep breaths, focusing on two at a time. You can use these to bring yourself fully present. With the first two breaths focus on releasing your body; inhale softness and exhale physical tension. Let your body sink deeply into the support you're resting on. The next two breaths are for quieting your thoughts. Let your mind become quiet. Release any extraneous thoughts, and bring your focus inward. Let the next two breaths open your heart; see or feel the warm light of your heart's love spill over and fill your whole body with warmth and compassion. Release any other emotions. With the next two breaths expand your awareness to your soul and your connection with Spirit, opening to the tenderness, love, and healing within you and surrounding you.

Allow your breathing to become easy and relaxed while you rest in the stillness and acceptance that encompasses your body, mind, heart, and soul. Again, let your body float on your breath, feeling it rise a bit on the in-breath, and settle with your out-breath. Let yourself feel grounded as if you have roots that extend down into the nourishing soil.

And now in your mind's eye, let yourself move to a special place, a place of comfort for you, beautiful and quiet, where you feel safe and peaceful. It may be a place where you've been before or it may be a new place. It can be real or imaginary, outdoors or inside. Just let yourself go there in your mind's eye. It doesn't matter where it is, as long as you feel peaceful and happy there. Explore this place in whatever way makes sense to you. Let yourself notice more and more about it, so that the image becomes richer and fuller, with more details. Look all around. Notice what you hear. Feel what the air feels like on your skin. Sense what time of day it is. And now notice where you would feel the most comfortable, and settle down in that spot. Let this place support you with its peaceful, healing presence.

And when you're ready, invite an image to form for your Inner Healer—a wise, loving figure, full of healing energy. Just allow an image to appear. Something in your special place may call itself to your attention as your healer; or it may be something that appears when you invite it to join you. The image can be something in nature, or a person, or a symbol. You may notice your healer when you look around your special place again, seeing something you hadn't noticed before. Whatever comes, welcome and accept this image of your healer. Notice everything you can about this healing image; become aware of size and shape, colors and textures. Notice any expression on your healer's features. Take a few moments and let this image become even clearer, noticing everything that makes it unique.

Be aware of your healer's love for you, the healing energy, and the deep wisdom; and if you find that the image is not unconditionally loving and accepting, thank it for coming, and for the intention to help, and let that image fade away; and invite another image that is full of healing, love, and wisdom.

You can pause the CD if you want more time for this.

And now, welcome your Healer in your own way, and let the image greet you in a way that you can understand. Let yourself feel your healer's acceptance and compassion for you. Become aware of the great healing power and ability to give you wise counsel. Now let our attention rest lightly on your question or concern about your health. Take some time to explore the issue with your healer. Allow your healer to respond in a way you can understand. Communicate back and forth in your own way to learn all you can about your concern. Let your healer deepen your understanding about your healing. And now notice if there's anything else you want to say or do with your Inner Healer before you close for today, and go ahead and do that.

Thank your inner healer for coming and sharing with you, knowing that you can return and meet with your healer again any time. Ask your healer to show you the easiest way to meet again, and if you want, set a time to do that. Now let your healing image go to wherever it will be until you meet in this way again. And now be aware of yourself resting in your peaceful place, remembering all you've learned and shared; and know that you'll bring back everything that's important.

And now let those images fade, and begin to bring your attention back to the external world around you. Be aware of the support you're resting on, and notice any sounds around you; begin to be aware of your body, all the way from your head down to your toes; move around a bit and stretch, to come fully present in your body. Allow the quiet, relaxed energy you've felt during this imagery to shift into a more invigorating, vitalizing kind of energy in your muscles and your body; and let your mind be alert and aware of all you're bringing back with you. When you're ready, open your eyes.

Appendix D: Talking with Your Pain–Exercise 12e
Script for Guided Self-Massage #4–KindTouch CD

Settle into a comfortable position and begin to turn your focus inward, allowing your eyes to gently close. Take a few deep breaths and let them be letting-go breaths. Let yourself float on your breath, feeling your body rise a bit when you inhale, and to settle with your exhalations.

I'll lead you through eight slow, deep breaths, focusing on two at a time. You can use these to bring yourself fully present. With the first two breaths focus on releasing your body, inhale softness and exhale physical tension. Let your body sink deeply into the support you're resting on. The next two breaths are for quieting your thoughts. Let your mind become quiet. Release any extraneous thoughts, and bring your focus inward. Let the next two breaths open your heart; see or feel the warm light of your heart's love spill over and fill your whole body with warmth and compassion. Release any other emotions. With the next two breaths expand your awareness to your soul and your connection with Spirit, opening to the tenderness, love, and healing within you and surrounding you.

Allow your breathing to become easy and relaxed while you rest in the stillness and acceptance that encompasses your body, mind, heart, and soul. Again, let your body float on your breath, feeling it rise a bit on the in-breath, and settle with your out-breath. Let yourself feel grounded as if you have roots that extend down into the nourishing soil.

And now in your mind's eye, let yourself move to a special place, a place of comfort for you, beautiful and quiet, where you feel safe and peaceful. It may be a place where you've been before or it may be a new place. It can be real or imaginary, outdoors or inside. Just let yourself go there in your mind's eye. It doesn't matter where it is, as long as you feel peaceful and happy there. Explore this place in whatever way makes sense to you. Let yourself notice more and more about it, so that the image becomes richer and fuller, with more details. Look all around. Notice what you hear. Feel what the air feels like on your skin. Sense what time of day it is.

And now notice where you would feel the most comfortable, and settle down in that spot. Let this place support you with its peaceful, healing presence.

And when you're ready, focus on the warm light in your heart, and from that energy, allow to appear in front of you, a sacred container or bowl. It can be anything, as long as it is shaped so that it can hold something. Explore this sacred container so that you notice everything about it – what it looks like, what it feels like to the touch. Now expand your awareness to sense how it is filled with compassion and tenderness, a place of safety. Let it glow with the richness of its love and healing presence. Let yourself be aware of resting in your peaceful, safe place with a sacred container of acceptance and compassion in front of you.

And now turn your attention inward, to a part of your body that is hurting or feels restricted. And without any effort, allow an image to arise for that pain or limitation. Just let the first image you notice emerge. And whatever it is, accept it without judgment, even if it makes no sense right now. Before exploring it further gently pick up this image for your pain or restriction and place it in the container in front of you. Let the sacred container hold this image of your pain with infinite understanding and compassion. And just take a minute to notice what happens.

And now that this image is resting in safety in front of you, notice everything you can about it. Notice its shape. Sense its size, and density. Notice its color and its textures. If it has feelings, notice them too. And sense what it is doing—is it resting, or doing something?

Now you'll have some time to communicate with this image of your pain. Ask it why it is here, and let it answer in a way you can understand; ask what it is trying to do for you.

And now, ask it what it needs from you; and really listen. This may be a message about a needed change in your life, or it may be a need your image has within the imagery world; either will help you, so be open to any message. If you want some help with this, invite your Inner Healer to join you; and ask for help in understanding.

If you want more time for this, pause the CD.

And now notice if there's anything else you want to say or do with this image of your pain or restriction before you close for today, and go ahead and do that.

And then thank it for coming and sharing with you; and release the image; and thank the sacred container for giving safety and compassion; and let it fade. If your Inner Healer joined you, express your gratitude for its help, and let this image go to wherever it will be until you meet in this way again; and now, just be aware of yourself resting in the beauty of your special place, gently thinking about what's just happened, knowing you'll bring back everything that's important.

And now let those images fade, and begin to bring your attention back to the external world around you. Be aware of the support you're resting on, and notice any sounds around you; begin to be aware of your body, all the way from your head down to your toes; move around a bit and stretch, to come fully present in your body. Allow the quiet, relaxed energy you've felt during this imagery to shift into a more invigorating, vitalizing kind of energy in your muscles and your body; and let your mind be alert and aware of all you're bringing back with you. And when you're ready, open your eyes.

Index

Index

About the Author

Lynne Walters earned a Bachelors Degree in Nursing from Stanford University and a Masters in Nursing from the University of Washington in Gerontological Nursing, the study of change and development through the adult life span. Lynne holds a national Holistic Nursing Certificate, HNC, a certificate in interactive guided imagery from the Academy for Guided Imagery, and one for Neuromuscular Massage Therapy. She has worked in hospice care, psychiatric nursing, home care nursing, and has led many workshops and classes in hospitals and in the community. In 1987 she started Whole Person Health Works, a private practice in holistic nursing and massage therapy.

Lynne's education in nursing (RN) and massage therapy (LMP) has been enhanced by several significant and chronic conditions that require her to listen to her body and heed its messages. This process has convinced her that physical problems can lead to more wholeness, not less, depending on how kindly we treat ourselves.

Lynne grew up in southern California, and wondered why she felt so dry all the time; she moved as soon as possible to the more invigorating, although wet, weather of the Pacific Northwest. Lynne and her husband live on an island in Puget Sound.